Body Massage for *Holistic* Therapists

Francesca Gould

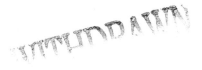
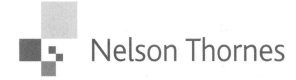

Nelson Thornes

Text © Francesca Gould 2004
Original illustrations © Nelson Thornes Ltd 2004

Published in 2004 by:
Nelson Thornes Ltd
Delta Place
27 Bath Road
CHELTENHAM
GL53 7TH
United Kingdom

09 10 11 12 / 10 9 8 7

A catalogue record for this book is available from the British Library

ISBN 978 0 7487 7654 2

Illustrations by Northern Phototypesetting Co Ltd, Bolton

Photography by Martin Sookias

Page make-up by Northern Phototypesetting Co Ltd, Bolton

Printed in China

Contents

Introduction

Massage is an extremely popular treatment and is carried out in many countries throughout the world. It can be defined as the 'manipulation of body tissues for therapeutic purposes'. Receiving a body massage brings numerous physical and emotional benefits.

This book mainly discusses Swedish massage techniques. It is specifically written for people undertaking professional massage courses, such as the VTCT Level 3 Certificate in Swedish Massage, VTCT Level 3 Diploma in Body Massage and ITEC Diploma in Body Massage. It is also useful as a reference tool for qualified students who wish to expand their knowledge of body massage.

Included in the book is a full body massage routine, where each massage movement is illustrated, as well as advanced massage techniques. In Chapter 2 you can label and colour in various parts of the body to help you expand your anatomy and physiology knowledge. There are also tasks and self-test questions throughout the book to test knowledge and help you to build a portfolio of evidence. The multiple choice questions will help you to prepare for examinations. The answers to the tasks and questions can be found – FREE – at *www.saloneducation.co.uk*.

Good luck!

Francesca Gould

April 2003

Acknowledgements

The author and publisher would like to thank the following people for their help with the production of this book:

The model Caroline Gammon for her support and professionalism; Martin Sookias for the wonderful photography; Ab Lagerholm UK (www.lagerholm.co.uk) for the photo on page 154; The Carlton Group for the photos on page 236; Heather Mole, Melanie Clague and Margaret Paul for reviewing the text.

Introduction to Massage 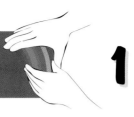 1

HISTORY OF MASSAGE

For thousands of years the laying on of hands or massage has been used to heal or comfort, and forms of massage are found in almost every culture. Holding or rubbing a part of the body that is causing discomfort is instinctive for humans.

China

Massage has been recorded in China from as early as 3000 BC. The Chinese found that applying pressure techniques was very effective on specific points on the body. These special techniques developed and became acupressure and acupuncture. These massage techniques spread to Japan where they were further developed and became known as shiatsu.

India

Massage is referred to in ancient Hindu books such as the 'Ayurveda' (Art of Life), which was written around 1800 BC. It describes how movements such as shampooing and rubbing were used to relieve tiredness, increase energy levels and improve general health.

Greeks and Romans

To the ancient Greek and Roman physicians, massage was one of the main ways of healing and relieving pain. Roman gladiators were vigorously massaged with oil to ensure their muscles were supple and warm before commencing battle. Around 1000 BC, the Greek poet Homer writes in the poem called 'The Odyssey' of Greek soldiers being rubbed and anointed with oils by beautiful women to aid their recovery and regain strength on return from battle.

The massage techniques used in Roman times included pummelling, pinching and squeezing. Every day Julius Caesar, who suffered from epilepsy, was pinched all over to help relieve his neuralgia and headaches.

Around 500 BC, Hippocrates, a Greek physician regarded as the father of medicine, regularly used massage on his patients to treat injury and disease. He wrote: 'The physician must be experienced in many things, but assuredly in rubbing … For rubbing can bind a joint that is too loose, and loosen a joint that is too rigid'. He also concluded that massage was more beneficial if the pressure was applied in an upward direction towards the heart.

Galen (AD 130–200), a Greek doctor, who had discovered that arteries contained blood and not air as was originally thought, recommended massage for treatment of injury and illness. He stated that massage strokes should be used in various directions according to the result required.

> **Note**
>
> Galen was the personal physician to the Roman Emperor Marcus Aurelius.

Arabs

After the fall of Rome in the fifth century AD, little is known about the use of massage until the eleventh century, when an Arab philosopher and physician called Avicenna noted that the object of massage was to disperse the effete (waste) matters found in the muscles. This would have helped to improve exhausted and weak muscles.

France

In the sixteenth century, a French doctor called Ambroise Pare (1517–90) graded massage into gentle, medium and vigorous. He used friction movements to help reduce swelling before treating dislocations of joints and is said to have successfully treated Mary Queen of Scots with massage.

Sweden

In the early 1800s, a Swedish physiologist called Per Henrik Ling (1776–1839) developed 'Swedish massage'.

He combined his knowledge of physiology, gymnastics, and Chinese, Egyptian, Roman and Greek massage techniques. He devised many of the massage movements used today, such as effleurage, petrissage, vibrations, rolling and slapping.

In 1813 the first college to offer Swedish massage was established in Stockholm, and it was later taught all over Europe. In 1894 a group of women founded the Society of Trained Masseuses and worked hard to raise standards and promote massage as a professional occupation. This later became the Chartered Society of Physiotherapy.

During both world wars massage was used to treat injured people, which led to a demand in trained therapists. Today, the demand for professional massage treatments continues to grow.

Task 1.1

Briefly describe the history of body massage in the table below:

	Brief history
China	
India	
Greeks and Romans	
Arabs	
France	
Sweden	

WHAT IS MASSAGE?

Massage is the manipulation of soft body tissue such as muscle and can be carried out manually or with machinery. The word 'massage' is thought to have derived from the Arabic word *mass'h*, meaning to press softly. In French *masser* means 'to rub' and in Greek *massein* means 'to knead'. The hands, thumbs, fingers, forearm or elbows can be used to apply pressure on to areas of the body. The massage movements in this book are based on the Swedish system of massage.

BENEFITS OF MASSAGE

There are numerous benefits of massage, both physical and emotional. These include the following:

- relaxes the mind and body
- increases the blood and lymphatic circulation, therefore brings oxygen and nutrients to the part being massaged and takes away waste products, which may be responsible for muscle stiffness, aches and pains
- relaxes tight muscles
- relieves stiff joints
- encourages deeper and relaxed breathing
- helps to induce feelings of calmness
- encourages sleep
- improves digestion
- improves condition of the skin
- creates feelings of well-being.

List the physical and emotional effects of body massage:

Physical	Emotional

STRESS

Massage treatment is helpful for stress-related problems. An understanding of stress and its causes will help you to treat the client holistically. For example, if your client is suffering from irritable bowel syndrome, probably due to stress, encourage the client to take time to relax. A change of lifestyle, such as taking up yoga and adopting a healthier diet or even developing a positive way of thinking, which will alleviate stress, can be advised.

Note

It is thought that over 70 per cent of all visits to the doctor are stress related.

Stress and its causes

Early man's survival depended on his skill at hunting and escaping predators. When under the threat of attack the body immediately reacts by releasing stress hormones. This is called the fight or flight response and has effects on the body such as increasing the heart rate, dilating the bronchioles, dilating the pupils, constricting the blood vessels of the skin and intestines, and dilating the blood vessels in the muscles. Stress is anything that triggers this fight or flight or adrenaline response.

Note

The term 'holistic' comes from the Greek word 'Holos' meaning whole.

Note

'Just for today do not anger, just for today do not worry.' Two of the Reiki principles.

We feel stressed when demands are placed on us and we do not feel we have the ability to cope with them. Sometimes these demands can be stimulating and we cope well, as we feel able to deal with them and in control of the situation. Stress is not necessarily a bad thing. It can help to motivate us and make us more effective and challenged.

Stress can be positive or negative. Positive stress could be described as a high, excited tension, e.g. when you are achieving success in your job. Performers, for example, experience this type of stress. Negative stress may be experienced while sitting behind the wheel of a car in a traffic queue. Other types of negative stress include bereavement, loss of a job, moving house, pregnancy, financial difficulties and break up of relationships.

People's personalities largely determine if they are likely to be vulnerable to the effects of stress. Competitive, ambitious over-achievers often tend to be stressed. These people can be impatient, hurried and highly conscious of time. People who are easygoing and calm are less likely to become stressed. They may often appear patient and relaxed.

Note

Integral biology is the study of the effects that our environment has on our health, e.g. our working environment, which may cause stress.

Many normally occurring stresses will be dealt with effectively by the body and we soon recover from them without any serious ill effect. Continual high stress levels cause an individual to become anxious and feel overloaded, until eventually exhaustion and burnout occur. When stress becomes excessive it affects every system of the body as well as the mind.

Men and women often respond differently to the effects of stress. Men are more likely to suffer from high blood pressure. However, women can become emotional and irritable, and suffer from headaches, irritable bowel syndrome, anxiety and depression. Stress is a contributory factor to almost every serious illness known to humanity. The more stressed you are the more likely you are to suffer from both physical and mental problems, which include:

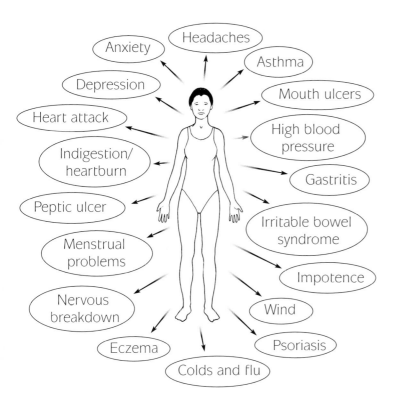

Figure 1.1 *Symptoms caused by stress*

General adaptation syndrome

Physiologist Hans Seyle used the term 'general-adaptation syndrome' (GAS) to describe the body's response to stress. He states that there are three phases:

1 The alarm reaction
The sympathetic nerves come into action as the body prepares for fight or flight. The increased flow of adrenaline (epinephrine) causes the heart to beat faster, the pulse and blood pressure to rise, and breathing to become quicker and shallower. There are also other physiological changes that happen when coping with an emergency situation. Symptoms include dizziness, sweating, churning stomach, nausea and poor sleeping

patterns. The adrenal glands release cortical and other key hormones into the bloodstream at this stage.

2 **The resistance stage**

This is when normal body functioning is disrupted, i.e. during the alarm reaction. The body strives for homeostasis, a state in which blood pressure, heart rate, hormone levels and other vital functions are maintained within a narrow range of normal. The resistance stage happens if stress continues over a long period of time, when blood pressure may remain high and stress-related illnesses might occur. Symptoms include high blood pressure, colds/flu, migraine, insomnia, eczema, depression, anxiety, and excessive smoking and drinking of alcohol.

3 **Exhaustion**

The body seems unable to make use of cortical hormones that are released from the adrenal cortex in response to stress. Burnout and exhaustion occur, and major organs become weakened and may function poorly.

Seyle has suggested that chronic stress is harmful to the body due to the side effects of long-term elevated levels of cortical hormones. The immune system does not work as efficiently so the body becomes susceptible to infections and there is strain put on the internal organs.

Massage can help reverse the effects of this stress cycle by calming the sympathetic nervous system, causing a reduction in the release of adrenaline. Massage also helps to slow down the heartbeat, lower the blood pressure and improve breathing. It reduces the symptoms of stress and anxiety, leaving people in a calmer and more relaxed state.

Advice to stress sufferers

The following advice can be given to someone suffering from negative stress:

- Do not dwell on past negative events. Free yourself to enjoy what is happening now.

- Become more assertive, learn to say NO.

- Turn negative thoughts into positive ones. Negative thoughts never did anyone any good.

- Worry only about the things you can control, not what you cannot.

- Become more organised and set regular, attainable goals. Tick them off as you achieve them.

- Writing things down often helps to clear anxieties and fears from the mind.

- Take up a hobby or some sort of activity such as yoga or t'ai chi. These are excellent for relaxation.

- Attend a stress management and relaxation course.

- Do not be afraid to ask for help and delegate responsibility to others.

Stress sufferers may overeat, undereat, smoke or drink a lot of alcohol. They should be encouraged to reduce caffeine, alcohol intake and also to stop smoking. This will help to limit the amount of toxins being put into the body, which will help the body to deal more effectively with the effects of stress. Diluted fruit or vegetable juices should be drunk in place of tea and coffee. These will supply vitamin C and magnesium. Both are important to maintain health, but are easily depleted when a person is stressed.

A healthy, well-balanced diet is very important and sufferers from stress should aim to eat a diet high in fruit and vegetables, wholegrain breads and cereals, and low in sugar and caffeine, to help give them a greater ability to cope. Certain nutrients have been shown to help deal with stress and support the organs that are involved in the stress reaction. Vitamins A, C and E, and the minerals zinc and selenium, are particularly recommended.

Note

It is advised to undertake a nutrition course before giving nutritional advice to clients.

The vitamin B group is largely responsible for the smooth running of the nervous system. A person depleted of vitamins B, C and zinc is also at increased risk of coming down with many minor infections such as colds, coughs, cold sores, etc.

Regular exercise such as walking, yoga and swimming is recommended. Exercise is a natural way to increase the release of endorphins, opiate-like substances that help to relieve pain and lift the mood.

Massage treatments are an excellent way of reducing stress and will not only help to relax the mind but also alleviate many of the physical symptoms of stress such as tense muscles, aching neck, shoulders and back.

HEALTHY BREATHING AND BREATHING EXERCISES

People use two types of breathing patterns. Upper-chest breathing lifts the chest upwards and outwards and the breathing tends to be shallow and rapid, such as during vigorous exercise. Relaxed or diaphragmatic breathing is deeper and slower; as the lower portions of the lungs are filled with air they push down on the diaphragm and cause the abdomen to protrude. For most people normal, everyday breathing tends to be mostly shallow and rapid.

Breathing is a powerful way to energise and relax the body. When done correctly it requires a person to inhale slowly and deeply through the nose and exhale through the mouth; this prevents the throat from becoming dry. As air is inhaled the stomach should be allowed to move outwards. The diaphragm is pulled downwards, causing the lungs to draw in air to fill the space. The diaphragm will then relax, causing air to be expelled from the lungs in an out breath.

Slow, deep and rhythmic breathing triggers a relaxation response in the body. Some of these changes include a slower heart rate, muscular relaxation and a feeling of calmness. Relaxation exercises will also trigger a relaxation response in the body.

Breathing exercise

1 *Stand with back straight and feet slightly apart.*

   Inhale slowly and deeply through the nose for about 4 seconds; think about bringing the breath into the abdomen. At the same time raise the arms backwards over the head.

2 *Momentarily hold the breath and then allow the arms and trunk to fall forwards.*

   (Ensure knees are bent to prevent any strain.) At the same time, breathe out, creating a 'Ha' sound.

3 *Breathe in slowly and deeply and slowly raise the body back into the standing position.*

   Repeat the exercise twice.

MEDITATION

Meditation has been part of many Eastern religions and philosophies. It involves calming the mind and will help encourage deep and clear thought and so aid concentration. It helps to relax tense muscles, lower blood pressure and regulate the breathing rate. Ensure the body is relaxed, warm and comfortable.

There are different ways to meditate, which can involve concentrating on a candle flame, a mark on the wall, the breathing pattern or words such as 'relax' or 'calm'.

If you choose to concentrate on a word such as 'calm', try to focus on this word only. Thoughts may pass through your head; acknowledge them and let them go by and continue to concentrate on the word 'calm'. Be aware of your breathing; ensure it is deep and slow.

During meditation a mantra, meaning speech, can help to focus the mind. The sound 'om' is often used and can be repeated with every exhalation.

Beginners who are unsupervised may find meditation difficult so it is advised they attend a yoga class or are supervised by someone who is experienced at meditation.

Meditative breathing exercise

This simple meditative breathing exercise will help to promote calm breathing.

1 **Sit comfortably with the eyes closed.**
Slowly breathe in and out through the nose. Concentrate on producing a long, deep, smooth exhalation. You will naturally inhale. Allow your breathing to settle into a smooth, regular rhythm.

2 **Relax your muscles.**
Visualise your thoughts as many bubbles and imagine all the bubbles floating away. You feel very warm and relaxed.

3 **Try to remain focused on your breathing.**
If other thoughts appear, acknowledge them and then let them float away in bubbles and again concentrate on your breathing.

4 **You will feel calm and relaxed.**
Practise this exercise for about 10 minutes every day.

RELAXATION EXERCISES

Relaxation exercises such as these can be beneficial to someone who is feeling stressed or anxious.

Exercise 1 Either sit or lie down and ensure you are comfortable. Breathing slowly and deeply, take in a deep breath as you carry out each hold and release movement.

Focus your attention on your feet, let your heels sink into the floor … floating … relaxing. Feel the tension running out of them. Clench the muscles of the lower legs, hold for about 5 seconds and then relax. They feel heavy and relaxed. Clench the muscles of the upper legs for about 5 seconds and then relax. Let the feeling of relaxation move up through the legs and flow through the hips and lower back … relaxing more with each breath. Clench the muscles of your buttocks and then relax them. Let your buttocks and pelvis sink into the floor … you feel very relaxed and comfortable … clench the muscles of your back and then relax them. Picture the muscles of the back becoming longer and wider. The body is feeling heavy and relaxed.

Let your shoulders relax. Tense the muscles of the chest and abdomen and then relax. Feelings of warmth and relaxation are running up through the body. Now tense the muscles in the arms, hold and release. They feel relaxed and floppy. Clench both hands into fist shapes, hold and release. Feel the tension draining out of the arms and hands. Let that feeling of comfort, warmth and relaxation move up to the face and head. Tense the muscles in the face and scalp, hold and then release. Your head feels heavy and relaxed. You feel very warm and comfortable. Your whole body feels heavy and relaxed. Floating … relaxing …

This exercise can be repeated twice. It is a good technique for releasing tension from muscles and so can help with headaches, aches and pains. It is excellent for relaxing the whole body.

Exercise 2 Close your eyes and take several deep breaths. Begin releasing tension in the neck by rolling the head slowly from side to side. Allow tension to drain from the head, face and neck like melting wax. Feel the tension flowing out of the chest and abdomen. Feel tension being released from the lower back and then upper back. Visualise all the tension being carried down through the

> **Note**
>
> Affirmations such as 'I feel relaxed' or 'I feel in control of my life' may be used during the relaxation exercises.

arms and out through the hands. Shake the hands to help rid this tension.

The whole upper body is now free of tension and feeling relaxed. Release tension from the buttocks and legs, continuing to breathe slowly. Imagine your legs are heavy and relaxed, and let your heels sink into the floor. Visualise the flow of tension running down the calves. Now, concentrate on your feet and think about how they feel. Imagine the tension and pressure of walking flowing out of the feet.

Now imagine a warm, healing light penetrating the top of your head and flowing through the body, down your arms and legs and out through the hands and feet, taking away all tension and troubling thoughts. This warm light is flowing freely around the body, helping to heal and relax the body.

VISUALISATION

Visualisation is a powerful tool for helping to de-stress and relax both you and your client. While carrying out the breathing or relaxation techniques you can imagine for example floating on a cloud or lying in a meadow. For the following exercise ensure the client's eyes are closed and that he or she is comfortable and warm.

Healing sanctuary

Imagine yourself walking along a beautiful secluded beach with golden sands. The sun is warm on your skin. You feel safe and very happy. There is a small boat floating on the calm turquoise sea, near the shore. You walk over to the boat. Any problems or negative thoughts you may have should be placed into the boat. When you have finished, gently push the boat out to sea and watch it float into the distance until it is no longer visible.

As you walk back up the beach you notice a small waterfall, the water droplets sparkling in the sunlight, gently cascading down. You can either walk through the waterfall or behind it; the water is cleansing, warm and fresh.

There is a secret place behind the waterfall: your healing sanctuary. Imagine a place that is beautiful and calming; only you know about this place. It can be a cave, room or whatever you like, but you feel contented, safe and relaxed. Visualise the contents of your sanctuary, by picturing anything that you would like. If you wish, you may have an angel there who protects you, listens to your fears and dreams, who hears you talk about your day and comforts you.

When you have had sufficient healing, walk back through the waterfall and along the beach…

Note

This visualisation would be an excellent way to prepare you prior to giving a massage.

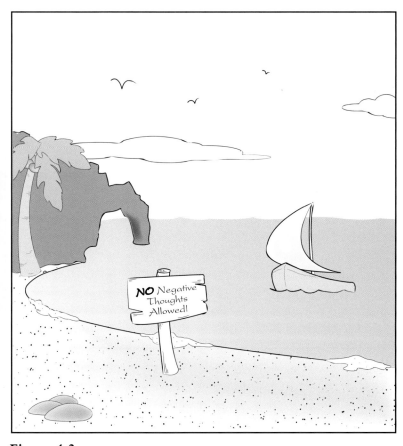

Figure 1.2

1. The word 'massage' is thought to have derived from which Arabic word meaning 'to press softly'?

   . . . .

2. Which Swedish physiologist developed Swedish massage?

   . . . .

3. State **3** benefits of massage.

   . . . .

   . . . .

   . . . .

4. Name **3** causes of negative stress.

   . . . .

   . . . .

   . . . .

5. State **5** physical or mental problems that are stress related.

   . . . .

   . . . .

   . . . .

   . . . .

   . . . .

6. What are the **3** phases of general adaptation syndrome?

....

....

....

7. State **3** pieces of advice that could be given to someone suffering from stress.

....

....

....

8. What dietary advice could be given to someone suffering from stress?

....

....

....

9. Name **3** beneficial responses that occur in the body when carrying out breathing and relaxation exercises.

....

....

....

10. What is the purpose of meditation?

....

....

....

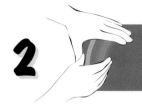

Body Systems and the Effects of Massage

This chapter gives a brief overview of the systems of the body and discusses the effects of massage. There are tasks throughout that require you to label and colour in diagrams.

CELLS AND TISSUES

Cells

Knowledge of the structure and function of cells will help you understand the systems of the body. Like the bricks of a house, cells are the building blocks of the body.

The body is made up of about 100,000 billion cells. Although tiny, cells are organised and complex structures. Different cells have certain functions, such as muscle, blood and fat cells, and can vary in size and shape. Groups of cells together make tissues and a group of tissues becomes an organ. A system is made up of various organs. Below is an example of the process:

1   Different types of **cells** make up the heart muscle;

2   many heart muscle cells together make up heart muscle **tissues**;

3   heart muscle tissues together make up the organ called the **heart**;

4   the heart is part of a **system** called the circulatory system.

Cell division (mitosis)

A cell does not keep on growing in size but will divide into two cells. The cells further multiply by splitting in half again and again to create tissues.

Epithelial and connective tissues

Epithelial tissues

Epithelial tissues form the coverings or linings of many organs and other structures in the body. There are two types of epithelial tissues: simple and compound. These tissues can be further subdivided as in the table below.

Table 2.1 Epithelial tissues

Simple	1	Pavement or squamous cells: these cells form the alveoli (air sacs) of the lungs, found in the lining of the heart, blood and lymph vessels
	2	Columnar cells: these cells line the ducts of most glands, the gall bladder and nearly the whole of the digestive tract
	3	Ciliated cells: these cells contain small hairs and line the respiratory passages, helping to prevent dust and bacteria from entering the lungs
Compound	1	Stratified epithelium: forms the top five layers of the skin and lines the mouth, throat, food pipe and anal canal
	2	Transitional epithelium: lines the bladder and ureters, helping to prevent rupture to organs, as this tissue is able to stretch

Connective tissues

Connective tissues may be solid, semi-solid or liquid. The main functions of these tissues include binding, support, transport, insulation and protection. There are various types of connective tissues, as listed in the table on page 20:

Table 2.2 Connective tissues

Areolar tissue	Areolar tissue is a thin, transparent tissue, which surrounds vessels such as blood vessels, nerves and muscle fibres in muscle. It also has the function of connecting the skin to muscles and other tissues.
Adipose tissue	Adipose tissue consists of fat cells. This fatty tissue is found in most parts of the body. It helps to support and protect organs, such as the kidneys.
Fibrous tissue	Fibrous tissue is made of collagen and is found in muscles, bones, tendons and ligaments.
Elastic tissue	Elastic tissue is found in walls of the arteries and in the air tubes of the respiratory tract where elasticity is needed.
Bone	Bone tissue consists of fibrous material, which gives the bone its strength.
Lymphoid	This tissue is found in lymph nodes. It is also found in the spleen, tonsils and appendix.
Cartilage	There are three types of cartilage found in the body: hyaline, elastic and fibro. Hyaline cartilage is found at joints. Elastic cartilage is found at the upper part of the ear. Fibro cartilage is found where great strength is required, such as the discs between the bones that form the spine.

Note

Blood is also a type of connective tissue.

SKIN

The skin provides a protective, waterproof covering over the whole body. It is made up of layers called the epidermis, dermis and subcutaneous layer.

Epidermis

The upper portion of the skin consists of five layers and is known as the epidermis; these are listed in Table 2.3 opposite.

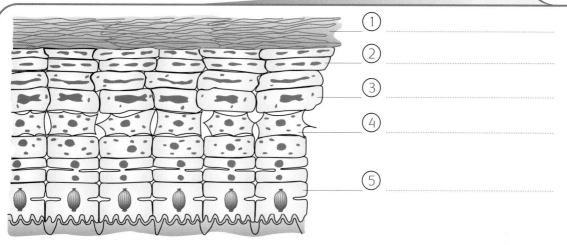

Figure 2.1 *Epidermis*

Label the diagram, matching the numbers to the numbered terms in Table 2.3. Use yellow shading for layers one and two. In layer three colour some cells yellow and some red. Colour layers four and five in red shading.

Table 2.3 Layers of the epidermis

Layer	Description
1 Horny layer (stratum corneum)	Top layer of epidermis. Consists of flat, overlapping dead cells. Cells are continually rubbed off the body by friction (desquamation) and replaced by cells from the layers beneath.
2 Clear layer (stratum lucidum)	Consists of dead cells. This layer is only found on fingertips, palms of hands and the soles of the feet.
3 Granular layer (stratum granulosum)	These cells have a granular appearance. The layer consists of living and dead cells. The living cells fill up with tiny granules, which causes them to die.
4 *Prickle cell layer* (stratum spinosum)	Cells are living and interlock by arm-like fine threads, giving the cells a prickly appearance. Pigment granules called melanin may be found here.
5 *Basal layer* (stratum germinatum)	Deepest layer and in contact with the dermis directly beneath it. The cells are living and divide (mitosis) to make new skin cells. As new cells are produced they push older cells above them towards the surface of the skin, until they finally reach the horny layer.

Skin pigmentation

Cells called melanocytes found within the basal layer produce granules of melanin. Melanin is responsible for the pigment (colour) of the skin and is stimulated by ultra-violet (UV) rays from the sun.

Dermis

Below the epidermis lies the dermis, which connects with the basal layer. It consists of two layers: the upper section is called the papillary layer and below it is the reticular layer. The dermis contains nerves, hair follicles, sebaceous glands, sweat glands and erector pili muscles.

The papillary layer contains small tubes called capillaries, which carry blood and lymph. This layer provides nutrients for the living layers of the epidermis. The reticular layer contains many connective tissue fibres. Collagen gives the skin strength and elastin gives the skin its elasticity.

The structures of the skin are described in Table 2.4 opposite.

Task 2.2

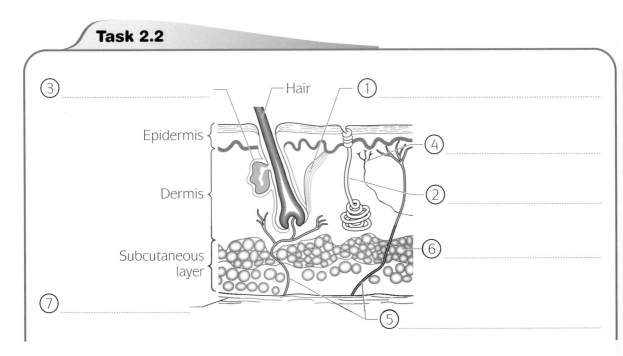

Figure 2.2 *Structures of the skin*

Label the diagram, matching the numbers to the numbered terms in Table 2.4. Use yellow shading to colour the sebaceous gland and adipose tissue, use red for the erector pili muscle, capillaries and muscle layer, and use blue for the nerve and sweat gland.

Table 2.4 The structures of the skin

Skin structure	Description and function
1 Erector pili muscles	Small muscles attached to the hair follicles. When cold, contraction of these muscles causes the hairs to stand on end, causing goose bumps. Air is trapped between the skin and hair and is warmed by the body heat, helping to keep the body warm.
2 Eccrine glands	Excrete sweat and are found all over the body. The sweat duct opens directly on to the surface of the skin through an opening called a pore. Sweat is a mixture of water, salt and toxins. Black skins contain larger and more numerous sweat glands than white skins.
3 Sebaceous glands	Small sac-like structures that produce sebum. This fatty substance is the skin's natural moisturiser. These glands are found all over the body. Hormones control the activity of these glands and as the body ages the secretion of sebum decreases causing the skin to become drier.
4 Sensory and motor nerve endings	Sensory nerve endings are found all over the body but are particularly numerous on our fingertips and lips. These nerves will make us aware of feelings of pain, touch, heat and cold by sending messages through sensory nerves to the brain. Messages are sent from the brain through motor nerves, which stimulate the sweat glands, erector pili muscles and sebaceous glands to carry out their functions.
5 Blood vessels	Blood within these vessels provides the skin with oxygen and nutrients. The living cells of the skin produce waste products such as carbon dioxide and metabolic waste. These waste products pass from the cells and enter into the bloodstream to be taken away and removed by the body.

Acid mantle

Sebum and sweat mix together on the skin to form an acid mantle. The acid mantle maintains the pH (acid/alkaline level) of the skin at 5.5–5.6 and this helps to protect the skin from harmful bacteria. Some soaps can affect the acid mantle and cause irritation and drying of the skin.

Subcutaneous layer

The subcutaneous layer is situated below the dermis. It consists of adipose tissue (fat) (6) and areolar tissue. The adipose tissue helps protect the body against injury and acts as an insulating layer against heat loss, helping to keep the body warm. The areolar tissue contains elastic fibres, making this layer stretchy and flexible. Muscle (7) is situated below the subcutaneous layer and is attached on to bone.

Functions of the skin

Table 2.5 discusses the functions of the skin.

Interesting facts about the skin

- Vitamin C is required by the body to produce collagen.
- Smoking causes a chemical to be released which destroys vitamin C.
- Long-term smokers are more prone to premature ageing of the skin than non-smokers.
- As the skin ages the collagen and elastin fibres break down, causing wrinkles and sagging of the skin.
- UV rays cause ageing of the skin and also damage the structure of the collagen and elastin fibres.
- Long-term use of hydrocortisone creams can cause thinning of the skin.
- While using antibiotics the skin can become dry.
- Pollution, such as exhaust fumes, can cause dehydration of the skin.

Table 2.5 The functions of the skin

Function of the skin		Description
Sensation		Sensory nerve endings send messages to the brain. These nerves respond to touch, pressure, pain, cold and heat and allow us to recognise objects from their feel and shape.
Heat regulation	Vasoconstriction	This occurs when the body becomes cold. The blood vessels constrict reducing the flow of blood through the capillaries. Heat lost from the surface of the skin is therefore reduced.
	Vasodilation	When the body becomes too hot the capillaries expand and the blood flow increases, allowing heat to be lost from the body by radiation.
	Goose bumps	Contraction of the erector pili muscles causes hairs to stand on end, keeping a layer of warm air close to the body.
	Shivering	Shivering helps warm the body, as the contraction of the muscles will produce heat.
	Sweating	Eccrine glands excrete sweat on to the skin surface; heat is lost as the water evaporates from the skin.
Absorption		The skin is largely waterproof and absorbs little, although certain substances can pass through the basal layer. Medications such as hormone replacement therapy can be given through patches placed on the skin. UV rays from the sun are also able to penetrate through to the basal layer.
Protection		Skin keeps harmful bacteria out and provides a covering for the organs inside. It protects the underlying structures from the harmful effects of UV light. The other functions of the skin also help to protect the body.
Excretion		Eccrine glands excrete sweat on to the skin's surface. Sweat consists of 99.4% water, 0.4% toxins and 0.2% salts.

→

Table 2.5 Continued

Function of the skin		Description
Secretion		Sebum is secreted from the sebaceous gland on to the skin's surface. It keeps the skin supple and helps to waterproof it.
Vitamin D		The UV rays from the sun penetrate through the skin's layers and activate a chemical in the skin, which changes into vitamin D. Vitamin D is essential for healthy bones and deficiency can cause rickets, a condition in which the bones are malformed.

SKIN DISEASES AND DISORDERS

Skin diseases and disorders can be classified as bacterial infections, viral infections, fungal infections, infestations, allergies and non-infectious conditions. As a therapist you are not expected to diagnose a skin condition; that is the job of a doctor. However, you need to be able to identify skin diseases and disorders that are contra-indicated to treatment, so that you do not worsen a condition or cross-infect.

Table 2.6 Bacterial infections

Bacterial infection	Brief description	Is it infectious and can affected area be massaged?
Boil	Inflamed pus-filled lump due to infection of the hair follicle. Often affects the back of the neck and armpits.	Infectious, so avoid the area during massage treatment.
Carbuncle	Group of boils involving several hair follicles.	Infectious, so avoid the area during massage treatment.
Impetigo	Weeping blisters, which form yellow coloured crusts. The surrounding area is red and inflamed. Common in children and usually found around the nose and mouth.	Infectious, so avoid the area during massage treatment. Clients should be referred to their doctor.

Table 2.7 Viral infections

Viral infection	Brief description	Is it infectious and can affected area be massaged?
Cold sore (herpes simplex virus)	Virus passes through the skin, travels up a nerve and lies dormant at a nerve junction. When stimulated by e.g. stress or sunlight it travels down the nerve and forms a cold sore. It begins as an area of redness, which blisters and forms a crust, usually around the mouth.	Highly infectious, so avoid the area during massage treatment.
Shingles (herpes zoster virus)	Caused by the chicken pox virus, which lies dormant in a nerve root and shows itself when the immune system is low. There are areas of redness and inflammation. It is itchy and blisters develop along nerve pathways, which then turn to crusty scabs.	Infectious, so no massage treatment should be given until the condition has cleared. Refer to a doctor.
Warts	An irregular growth appears above the surface of the skin. Mainly occur on the hands and can be itchy and painful. They often disappear after about a year without treatment.	Infectious, so the area should be avoided during massage treatment.
Verrucae	Warts that appear on the soles of the feet and contain black speckling.	Infectious, so the area should be avoided during massage treatment.

Table 2.8   Fungal infections

Fungal infection	Brief description	Is it infectious and can affected area be massaged?
Athlete's foot	Mostly affects areas between the toes and sole of the foot. Skin is cracked and itchy with flaking pieces of dead white skin. Skin may be sore and swollen and blisters may form.	It is highly infectious and the affected area must be avoided during treatment.
Ringworm	Red, scaly circular patches, which spread outwards. Centre of patch heals, forming a ring shape. Sometimes caught through touching animals.	Highly infectious, so area must be avoided during massage treatment.

Table 2.9   Infestations

Infestation	Brief description	Is it infectious and can the affected area be massaged?
Scabies	Mites burrow into the skin and lay eggs. Wavy, greyish lines can be seen commonly in webs of the fingers and crease of the elbow. It is very itchy with red lumps.	Highly infectious, so no massage treatment should be given and clients should consult their doctor.
Hair lice	Blood-sucking parasite lives in hair and lays eggs, white or yellowish in colour, which attach to the hair. Causes redness and itching.	Highly infectious, so no massage treatment should be given.

Table 2.10 Pigmentation disorders

Pigmentation disorders	Brief description	Is it infectious and can affected area be massaged?
Chloasma	Areas of darkened skin, often seen on the face. May be due to sunburn, pregnancy or contraceptive pill.	It is not infectious and the affected area can be massaged.
Vitiligo	Complete loss of colour in areas of the skin. Cause is unknown. Affected areas are very sensitive to sunlight and burn easily.	It is not infectious and the affected area can be massaged.

Table 2.11 Skin allergies

Skin allergy	Brief description	Is it infectious and can affected area be massaged?
Allergies	An abnormal response by body's immune system to a particular substance. Skin becomes warm, red and swollen.	It is not infectious but the affected area should be avoided during massage.
Urticaria	Also called nettle rash or hives. An allergic reaction that causes itchy lumps that are whitish with a red inflamed area around them. Causes include certain foods, drugs and stress.	It is not infectious but the affected area should be avoided during massage treatment. If the eyes, lips or throat are affected, seek medical attention as breathing may be impaired.
Dermatitis	Inflammation and redness of the skin due to external irritants such as detergents. There may also be itching and flaking of the skin.	It is not infectious but it is advisable not to work over the affected area, especially if there is bleeding and if the client feels discomfort.
Eczema	Inflammation of the skin and itchy, dry, scaly, red patches. Often affects creases of elbows and knees, also armpits. Small blisters may burst causing the skin to weep. Causes include detergents, cosmetics, stress and dairy products.	It is not infectious but it is advisable to avoid the affected area during massage treatment, especially if there is bleeding and weeping and if the client feels discomfort.

Table 2.12 Sebaceous gland disorders

Sebaceous gland disorder	Brief description	Is it infectious and can affected area be massaged?
Milia (whiteheads)	Dead skin cells cover the opening of hair follicle and causes sebum to become trapped. A milium can be seen as a small white spot and often accompanies dry skin.	It is not infectious and the affected area can be massaged.
Comedomes (blackheads)	Can be seen as black dots on the skin. They occur when sebum becomes trapped in the hair follicle. On exposure to air, the oil blackens due to oxidation. Generally accompanies greasy skin types.	It is not infectious so the affected area can be massaged.
Acne vulgaris	Red and swollen spots appear mainly on the face, neck and back. Caused by over-production of sebum. Sebum and dead skin cells become trapped causing spots to form.	It is not infectious but it is advisable to avoid the area during massage or obtain the advice of a doctor.
Acne rosacea	More common in women and mainly affects people over 30. The nose, cheeks and forehead appear flushed and reddened, producing a butterfly shape. Skin may become lumpy and pus-filled spots may appear.	It is not infectious but care needs to be taken when massaging over the affected areas. Avoid massage if there is any bleeding or if the client feels any discomfort.

Table 2.13 Abnormal skin growth conditions

Abnormal skin growth condition	Brief description	Is it infectious and can affected area be massaged?
Psoriasis	Skin cells reproduce too quickly causing thickened patches of skin that are red, dry, itchy and covered in silvery scales. Can affect any part of the body. Cause is unknown, although hereditary factors and stress play a part.	It is not infectious so massage treatment can be given providing there is no bleeding or weeping and the client does not feel any discomfort.
Skin tag	Loose, fibrous tissue that protrudes from the skin and is mainly brown in colour.	It is not infectious but it is advisable to avoid affected area during massage treatment as it may be uncomfortable for the client.
Corn	Thickening of horny layer of the skin mostly found on the joints of the toes. Can be quite painful. Can be caused by tight shoes.	It is not infectious but the affected area should be avoided during massage treatment to avoid discomfort.
Basal and squamous cell carcinomas	Account for 95% of all skin cancers. Usually found on areas of the body exposed to the sun. Begin as small, shiny, rounded lumps and form into ulcers. Brought on by UV light and usually found in fair-skinned people.	It is not infectious but obviously the area should be avoided during massage. The advice of a doctor should be sought.
Melanoma	A skin growth due to over-activity of the melanocytes caused by excessive exposure to the sun. Often occur at site of a mole. Although rare it is extremely dangerous. It is irregular in outline, patchy in colour, itchy or sore and may bleed.	It is not infectious but should obviously be avoided during massage treatment. The advice of a doctor should be sought.

Note

Never mention to the client that a lump may be malignant!

Effects of massage on the skin

- The circulation is improved and so fresh blood brings nutrients to the sebaceous glands; therefore sebum production is increased. More sebum helps to make the skin soft and supple.

- The sweat glands become more active and so more sweat is excreted. Toxins such as urea and other waste products are eliminated from the body in this way.

- Massage also causes the top layer of dead skin cells to be shed (desquamation), which improves the condition of the skin, giving it a healthy glow.

- The sensory nerve endings can either be soothed or stimulated, depending on the massage movements used.

SKELETAL SYSTEM

The skeletal system consists of the bones and joints of the body. There are 206 bones in the human body, which continue to grow up to the ages of between 18 and 25. After 25 the bones stop growing, although they can still continue to thicken.

Bone is living tissue and is constantly being built up and broken down. It is made up of 30 per cent living tissue such as collagen and 70 per cent minerals and water. The minerals include mainly calcium and phosphorus. A tough fibrous membrane called the periosteum, which is made up of two layers, covers the bones. The inner layer produces new cells for the growth and repair of the bone tissue, and the outer layer contains a rich blood supply, which provides nutrients for the bone.

Functions of the skeleton

The functions of the skeleton are discussed in Table 2.14 opposite.

Table 2.14 Functions of the skeleton

Function	Description
Shape/support	The skeleton gives the body its shape and supports the weight of all the other tissues.
Attachment for muscles and tendons	Bones provide the attachment point for the tendons of most skeletal muscles.
Development of blood cells	Red blood cells, white blood cells and platelets are produced within the red bone marrow of the bone.
Protection	Bones help to protect vital organs from injury, e.g. the ribs protect the heart and lungs and the skull protects the brain.
Movement	When skeletal muscles contract, they pull on bones to produce a movement.
Mineral store	Bones store the minerals calcium and phosphorus, which are important for the strength of the bone.

Regular exercise is essential as it not only prevents loss of bone but also stimulates the formation of new, stronger bone tissue. Bones adapt to the stress of exercise by laying down more calcium and other minerals, and also increase the amount of collagen fibres.

Ligaments

Ligaments consist of bands of strong, fibrous connective tissue, which are silvery in appearance. They prevent dislocation by holding the bones together across joints, but stretch slightly to allow movement.

Tendons

Tendons consist of white, strong, almost inelastic, fibrous bands. Most muscles are attached to bones by tendons. They vary in length and thickness. When a muscle contracts, the force transmitted through the tendon creates movement at the bone. An example of a tendon is the Achilles tendon that attaches the calf muscle to the heel.

Note

Ligaments and tendons have a poor blood supply so when they are damaged they can take a while to heal.

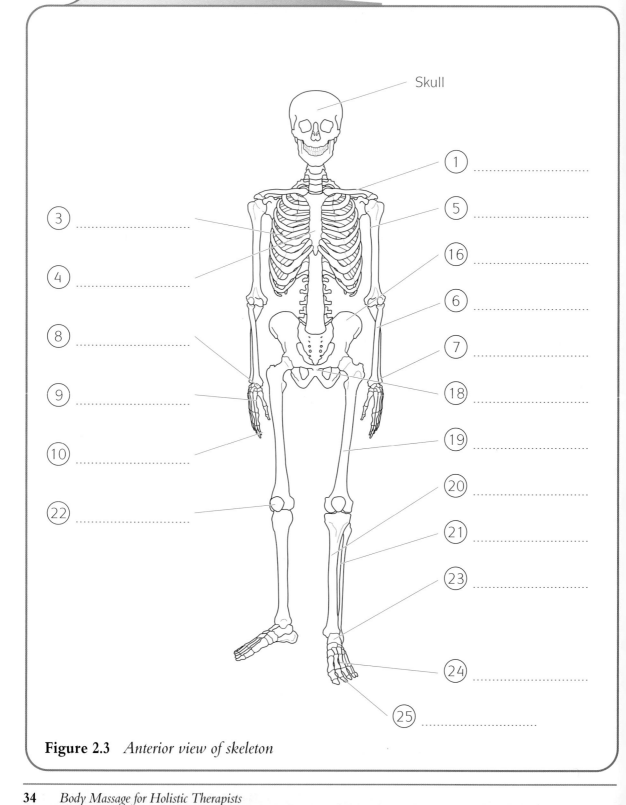

Skull

Figure 2.3 *Anterior view of skeleton*

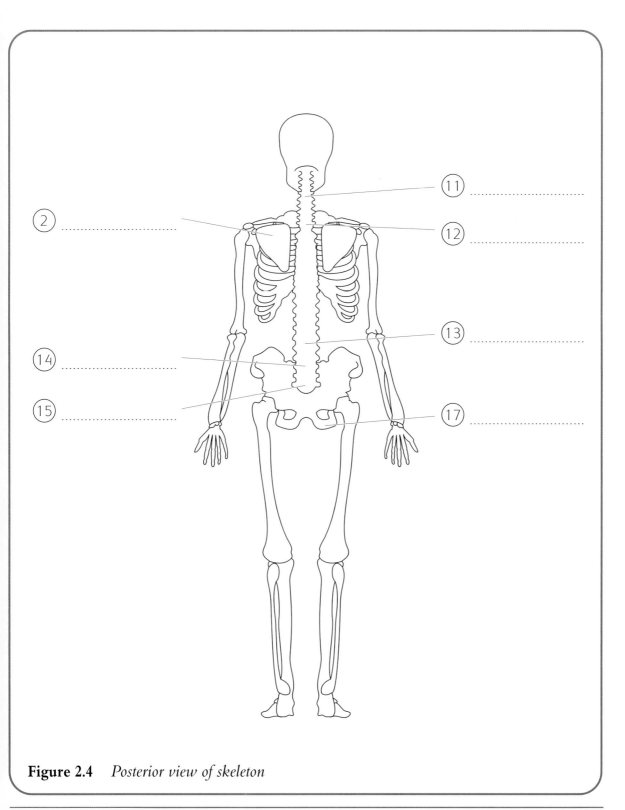

Figure 2.4   *Posterior view of skeleton*

Label the diagrams using the information below. Use yellow shading to colour the bones of the skeleton.

Bones of the shoulder girdle

1 **Clavicle:** a long, slender bone also known as the collar bone, of which there are two

2 **Scapula:** a large, triangular, flat bone also known as the shoulder blade, of which there are two

Thorax: the thoracic cavity (chest) contains organs such as the heart and lungs, which are protected by the ribcage.

3 **Ribs:** there are 12 pairs of ribs

4 **Sternum**: one bone, also known as the breast bone

Upper limbs

5 **Humerus:** long bone of the upper arm

6 **Radius:** situated on the thumb side of the forearm

7 **Ulna:** situated on little finger side of the forearm

8 **Carpals:** consist of eight small bones in the wrist

9 **Metacarpals:** consist of five metacarpal bones (long bones), which form the palm of the hand

10 **Phalanges:** the bones of the fingers, of which there are 14. One of these bones is known as a phalanx.

Vertebral column (spine): supports the upper body and encloses and protects the spinal cord. It consists of 33 bones, which are divided into five groups known as cervical, thoracic, lumbar, sacrum and coccyx.

11 **Cervical:** consists of seven vertebrae

12 **Thoracic:** consists of 12 vertebrae

13 **Lumbar:** consists of five bones and are the largest vertebrae

14 **Sacrum:** consists of five vertebrae fused together

15 **Coccyx:** consists of four bones fused together
= 33 bones

Note

There are 12 pairs of ribs and 12 thoracic vertebrae.

Intervertebral discs: in between the bones of the spine are pads of white fibrocartilage known as intervertebral discs. The intervertebral discs are thicker in the lumbar region than in the cervical region and are kept in place by ligaments. Their functions are to act as shock absorbers and to give the spine some flexibility so movement can be made.

Pelvic girdle: the pelvic girdle consists of three bones fused together

16 **Ilium:** the largest of the three bones. The iliac crest can be felt by placing the hand on the hip

17 **Ischium:** forms the posterior aspect of the pelvis

18 **Pubis:** situated on the anterior aspect of the pelvis

Note

The female's pelvis is wider and shallower and so has more space than the male's. This is due to the requirements of pregnancy and childbirth.

Bones of the lower limbs

19 **Femur:** the thigh bone and the longest bone in the body

20 **Tibia:** situated on anterior aspect of lower leg, also known as the shin bone

21 **Fibula:** situated on the lateral side to the tibia and thinner than the tibia

22 **Patella:** kneecap, articulates (joins) with the femur

23 **Tarsals:** there are seven tarsal (ankle) bones, which form the posterior part of the foot

24 **Metatarsals:** there are five metatarsal bones in the foot

25 **Phalanges:** there are 14 phalanges, which form the toes

Arches of the feet

The bones of the feet make up a bridge-like structure. The feet have three main arches, the shape of which is maintained by the bones, ligaments and muscles of the feet.

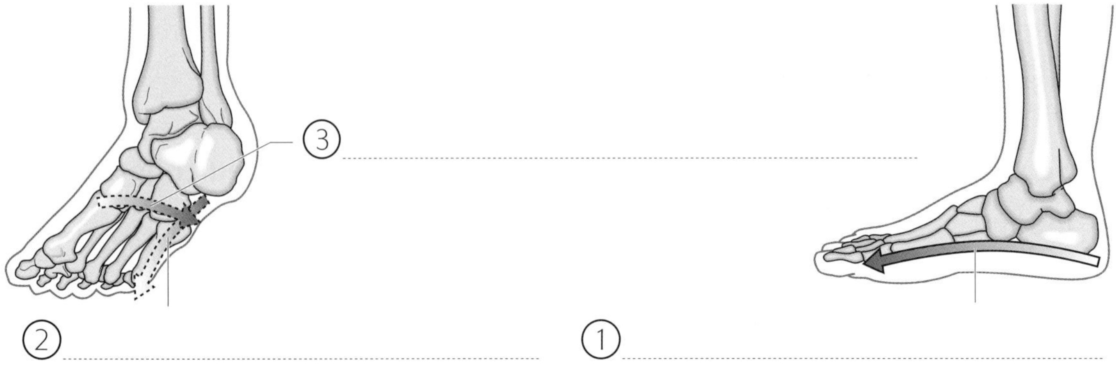

Figure 2.5 *Arches of the feet*

Label the diagram using the information below:

1 The **medial longitudinal arch** is the highest arch on the big toe side of the foot

2 The **lateral longitudinal arch** is found on the little toe side of the foot

3 The **transverse arch** runs across the foot

Note

Flat feet are due to fallen medial arches and exercises such as picking up marbles with the toes help to build up these arches.

Joints of the body

A joint describes the joining (articulation) of two or more bones of the body. There are three main types: fibrous (immovable), cartilaginous (slightly movable) and synovial (freely movable).

- **Fibrous** or immovable joints are fixed joints in which no movement between the joints is possible. Examples are the sutures or joints between the skull bones.

- **Cartilaginous** joints are slightly movable joints in which only limited motion is possible. Examples are bones of the vertebral column with their intervertebral discs of fibrocartilage.

- **Synovial** joints are freely movable joints of which there are several types, all having similar characteristics. An example is the joint of the knee.

Note

The midline is an imaginary line that runs through the middle of the body from the head and through the trunk.

Joint movements

Joints allow several different types of movement to be made. There are some basic terms used to describe these movements, shown in Table 2.15 below.

Table 2.15   Joint movement

Joint movement	Description
Flexion	A movement in which the body part bends and there is a decrease in the angle between the bones.
Extension	The opposite of flexion. The angle between the bones increases and the body part straightens.
Adduction	Movement towards the midline of the body.
Abduction	Movement away from the midline of the body.
Rotation	The rotary movement of bone around its axis.
Circumduction	A circular movement.
Supination	Rotating the arm, turning the palm of the hand to face outwards.
Pronation	Rotating the forearm, turning the palm to face inwards.
Inversion	Inward movement of the foot towards the midline.
Eversion	Outward movement of the foot away from the midline.

Task 2.5

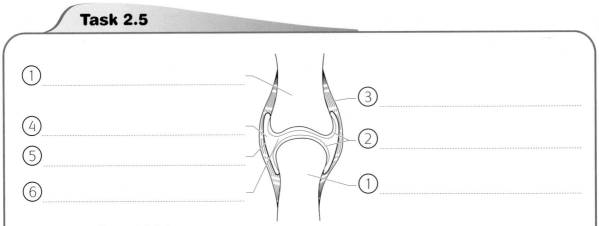

Figure 2.6 *Synovial joint*

Label and colour in the diagram in Figure 2.6 using the information below. Leave the bones unshaded. Use brown shading for the hyaline cartilage, grey shading for the ligaments and yellow shading for the synovial fluid.

In a freely movable joint ends of the **bones** (1) are mostly covered by **hyaline cartilage** (2). The cartilage helps to reduce friction and act as a shock absorber during movement. **Ligaments** (3) are needed to bind the bones together and help prevent dislocation. The space between the bones is called the **joint cavity** (4) and is enclosed by a capsule of fibrous tissue. The **synovial membrane** (5) lines the joint cavity and secretes a fluid called **synovial fluid** (6), which lubricates the joint and provides the hyaline cartilage with nutrients.

Various types of synovial joint are discussed in Table 2.16 opposite.

Table 2.16 Synovial joints

Synovial joint	Description	Joint movement
Ball and socket joint Examples are the shoulder and hip joints.	A rounded head of a bone fits into a cup-shaped cavity.	Flexion, extension, adduction, abduction, rotation and circumduction.
Hinge joint Examples are elbow and knee joints.	A round surface fits into the hollow surface of another bone.	Extension and flexion.
Saddle (or condyloid) joints Examples include joints in the wrist between the radius and ulna and between the skull and lower jaw.	This joint is similar to a hinge joint, but allows more movement.	Flexion, extension, abduction, adduction and slight circumduction.
Pivot joint An example is the radius, which rotates around the ulna at the elbow.	A socket in one bone rotates around a peg on another.	Rotation, supination and pronation.
Gliding joint Examples are the joints between the carpals and tarsals.	Two flat surfaces of bone glide over each other.	Flexion, extension, eversion and inversion.

Effects of massage on the skeleton and joints

A layer of connective tissue called the periosteum covers bones. Blood vessels from the periosteum penetrate the bone, providing the bone with nutrients. Deep massage movements stimulate blood flow to the periosteum and so increase the supply of nutrients to the bone.

Joints are nourished as the increased blood supply to the area brings oxygen and nutrients. Massage also helps to ease stiff joints and loosen adhesions such as scar tissue in structures around joints. For example, frictions across a ligament help to loosen it from underlying structures.

Sprain

Wrenching or twisting a joint, causing injury to its ligaments, can cause a sprain. It occurs when ligaments are stressed beyond their normal capacity.

Arthritis

The term 'arthritis' refers to many different diseases, most of which are characterised by inflammation of one or more joints. Pain and stiffness may also be present in muscles near the joint. The two main kinds are osteoarthritis and rheumatoid arthritis. Osteoarthritis is the most common form of arthritis. It often affects people who have been used to vigorous exercise and have worn the lining of their joints away. Rheumatoid arthritis is the more severe form of arthritis and will affect one person in a hundred. It occurs when the membrane that lines the joint becomes thick and swollen, and usually affects the fingers and toes first.

Bursitis

Some synovial joints contain a sac-like structure called a bursa, which helps to provide padding where tendons rub against bones or other tendons. Bursitis is inflammation of the bursa. Examples include tennis elbow, housemaid's knee and bursitis of the shoulders.

MUSCULAR SYSTEM

There are over 600 muscles in the body, which make up 40 to 50 per cent of the body weight. The function of the muscles is to produce movement, maintain posture and provide heat for the body.

The muscular system comprises three types of muscles: involuntary, cardiac and voluntary.

Involuntary muscle, also known as smooth muscle, is not under our conscious control. Smooth muscle makes up the walls of the blood and lymph vessels along with other vessels. The muscles allow the walls to relax and constrict.

The cardiac muscle is specialised tissue found only in the heart. This muscle never tires, indeed if it does we have serious problems.

Massage therapists are mostly concerned with voluntary muscles, also known as skeletal muscles, which are under our conscious control. Skeletal muscles consist of bundles of muscle fibres, which are striped in appearance and enclosed in a sheath (fascia). They allow movement of the body. Each person is born with a set amount of muscle fibres. Exercise will cause the individual muscle fibres to increase in size and so the muscle becomes larger.

Skeletal muscles are richly supplied with blood vessels and nerves. Before movement of a muscle can occur a message must be sent from the brain through a motor nerve, which will in turn stimulate the muscle to contract. The point at which a motor nerve enters a muscle is called the motor point. A motor nerve branches out, the ends of which are called motor end plates and rest on muscle fibres. Each muscle fibre will have its own nerve ending. Branches of one motor nerve can stimulate up to 150 muscle fibres at any one time.

Muscles are covered in fibrous tissue called fascia; this sheath extends to become tendons and attaches the muscle to bone. Fascia allows the muscles to glide smoothly past each other but will sometimes adhere to each other. The affected muscles will not function as well so there may be restricted movement and some discomfort. Massage will help to loosen the fascia so that the muscles no longer stick to each other and can once again glide smoothly.

Skeletal muscles bring about movement by exerting a pull on tendons, which cause the bones to move at the joints. The pulling force that causes movement is due to contraction (shortening) of the muscle.

Note

Strains to the fascia can lead to the formation of scar tissue.

Muscle tone

Muscle is never completely at rest, but always partially contracted. The partial contraction is not enough to move the muscle but will cause some tension. All skeletal muscles must be slightly contracted if the body is to remain upright. If all of the muscles relaxed then the body would fall to the floor. This continuous slight tension is involuntary and is known as muscle tone. Different groups of muscle fibres contract at different times, preventing the muscle becoming fatigued.

Each person's degree of muscle tone will vary depending on the amount of activity or exercise taken. People who do not exercise usually have poor muscle tone, as the muscle fibres do not contract as far as they should. This results in a lowering of muscle tone and so the muscles are said to be flaccid. Muscles with high degree of tone are called spastic as they are hard and rigid due to over-contraction. This can be seen in body-builders. Regular exercise and massage can help to maintain the elasticity of the muscle fibres, which will improve the tone of the muscle.

Muscle fatigue

Muscles require fuel in the form of glucose, and oxygen is needed to burn the glucose to make energy. When muscles become overworked, such as during vigorous exercise, the oxygen and glucose supplies are used up. If there is insufficient oxygen and glucose the muscles cannot produce enough energy to contract. The contractions will become weaker until they eventually stop. This is known as muscle fatigue.

As a result of muscle fatigue an accumulation of harmful waste products such as lactic acid and carbon dioxide start to build up in the affected muscle, causing stiffness and pain. Muscle fatigue is common among athletes who compete in endurance sports such as marathon races. Resting and gentle massage of the muscle will ensure the blood brings oxygen and glucose, and removes the waste products so that the muscles can work properly again.

Muscle strain

Overwork or over-stretching of the muscles can cause strain and may result in muscle fibres being torn. It can normally be felt as hardness in the muscle, which usually runs the same way as muscle fibres.

Tearing of muscle fibres

Injury to a muscle can cause complete or partial tearing of the muscle fibres. Partial tears result in the tearing of some muscle fibres and will feel very tender and painful, especially when contracting the muscle. Complete tearing involves tearing of all the muscle fibres, which causes the two ends of the muscles to contract away from each other. This is extremely painful and there is complete loss of function.

Adhesions and fibrous tissue

Injury and damage to the muscle may cause scar tissue to form due to insufficient healing by collagen fibres, perhaps because the muscle remained tense while healing took place. The scar tissue creates adhesions and fibrous tissue. Muscle fibres need to be able to glide smoothly past each other, but cannot do this when the fibres are stuck together (adhesions). After a while the fibres will knit together and form a hard lump or **knot** (fibrous tissue). Massage will help separate the fibres so they can continue to slide past each other, therefore restoring function to the muscle.

Note

Vigorous exercise can cause minor tearing of muscle fibres and is thought to be a major factor in why muscles become sore and stiff 12 to 48 hours afterwards.

Cramp

Cramp is a painful muscle spasm that may arise following exercise. Muscle spasms occur when muscles contract for too long, or when excessive sweating causes water and salt loss. The accumulation of lactic acid in the muscles following vigorous exercise may also cause cramp. Lightly massaging and gradually stretching the affected muscle can relieve the spasm and pain. Sometimes cramp can occur for no reason, such as during sleep, and may be due to poor muscle tone. It is also common during pregnancy.

Origin and insertion

The origin of the muscle is the bone to which it is attached, and this does not move. The insertion is the bone to which the muscle is attached and this does move, e.g. the bicep of the upper arm has its point of origin at the shoulder, while the point of insertion is the radius of the lower arm. The insertion is the part furthest away from the spine. Muscles always move towards their origins.

Muscles in the body normally work in pairs to produce movement. During movement one muscle will contract while another relaxes.

The muscle or muscles that move and contract are known as the prime mover(s). The muscle or muscles that relax

Note

All of the muscles that are responsible for backward movements are to be found at the back of the body and all of the muscles concerned with forward bending are found at the front of the body. This will help you to remember the actions of the muscles.

while the prime mover is contracting are known as the antagonist(s).

For example, when we bend a forearm, the muscle at the front of the arm (biceps) contracts so is called the prime mover. The muscle at the back of the arm (triceps) relaxes so is known as the antagonist.

Anatomical terms

To understand the terms listed in Table 2.17 the body has to be in the correct anatomical position. The body stands erect with arms by the side and palms facing forwards. There is an imaginary vertical line that runs through the middle of the body from the head and through the trunk. It is known as the midlinc.

Table 2.17 Anatomical terms

Anatomical term	Description
Medial	Nearer to the midline of the body. The ulna is on the medial side of the forearm.
Lateral	Towards the outer side or further away from the midline of the body. The humerus is lateral to the clavicle.
Anterior or ventral	Nearer to or at the front of the body. The sternum is anterior to the heart.
Posterior or dorsal	Nearer to or at the back of the body. The heart is posterior to the sternum.
Plantar	On or towards the sole of the foot.
Superficial	Towards the surface of the body. The skin is superficial to the heart.
Deep	Away from the surface of the body. The heart is deep to the skin.

Muscles of the body

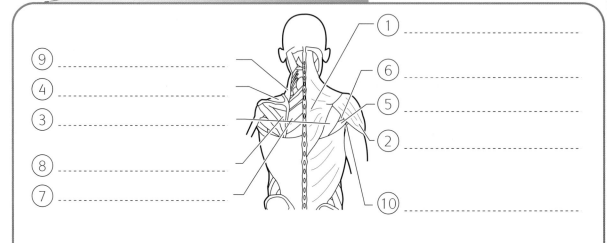

Front of body   Back of body

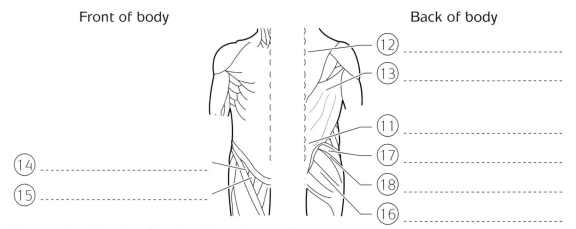

Figure 2.7   *Muscles of the shoulders, back and pelvis*

Label and colour in the diagram using the information given over the next few pages. Colour the muscles of the shoulders and back in red, and the bones and tendons in yellow.

Note

Shade lightly when colouring the muscles and ensure you use strokes that follow the direction of muscle fibres. It is important to understand the direction of these fibres when massaging.

Muscles of the shoulders

1 Trapezius
Position: superficial muscle that forms a large, kite-shaped muscle across the top of the back and neck
Origin: occipital bone and vertebrae
Insertion: scapula and clavicle
Action: lifts the clavicle as in shrugging and also draws the head backwards

2 Deltoid
Position: superficial, thick muscle that is triangular in shape and caps the shoulder
Origin: clavicle and scapula
Insertion: humerus
Action: abducts the arm, and draws it backwards and forwards

3 Infraspinalis
Position: deep muscle that covers the lower part of the scapula
Origin: scapula
Insertion: humerus
Action: laterally rotates and adducts arm

4 Supraspinalis
Position: deep muscle that covers the upper part of the scapula
Origin: scapula
Insertion: humerus
Action: helps deltoid muscle to abduct arm

5 Teres major
Position: deep muscle across back of shoulders
Origin: scapula
Insertion: humerus
Action: helps medially rotate and adduct arm

6 Teres minor

Position: deep muscle, across back of shoulders
Origin: scapula
Insertion: humerus
Action: laterally rotates and adducts arm

7 Rhomboids

Position: between vertebral column and scapula
Origin: thoracic vertebrae
Insertion: scapula
Action: rotates and adducts (pulls) scapula towards spine

8 Subscapularis

Position: large, triangular muscle found beneath scapula
Origin: scapula
Insertion: humerus
Action: medially rotates arm

9 Levator scapula

Position: deep muscle found at back and side of neck, on to scapula
Origin: cervical vertebrae
Insertion: scapula
Action: lifts shoulder and scapula

10 Coraco-brachialis

Position: upper medial part of arm
Origin: scapula
Insertion: humerus
Action: flexes and adducts arm

Muscles of the posterior aspect of trunk and pelvis

11 Quadratus lumborum
Position: deep muscle found medially on lower part of the back
Origin: iliac crest
Insertion: ribs
Action: lateral flexion (side bending) of lumbar vertebrae, assists diaphragm when breathing in

12 Erector spinae
Position: three groups of muscles found either side of vertebrae
Origin: vertebrae, ribs, iliac crest
Insertion: cervical and lumbar vertebrae, ribs
Action: extends the spine and so helps to hold the body in an upright position

13 Latissimus dorsi
Position: superficial, large sheet of muscle down back of lower thorax and lumbar region
Origin: vertebrae
Insertion: humerus
Action: draws the arm back and inwards towards the body. Help to pull body upwards when climbing

14 Psoas
Position: muscle found in lumbar region of spine and across hip joint
Origin: lumbar vertebrae
Insertion: femur
Action: together with iliacus, flexes thigh and helps to laterally rotate thigh

15 Iliacus

Position: muscle of the pelvis that crosses hip joint
Origin: ilium
Insertion: femur
Action: together with psoas, flexes thigh and helps to laterally rotate thigh

16 Gluteus maximus

Position: superficial muscle found in lower part of back forming buttocks
Origin: ilium, sacrum, coccyx
Insertion: femur
Action: extends the hip and rotates thigh laterally, used in running and jumping

17 Gluteus medius

Position: lateral part of buttocks, deep to gluteus maximus
Origin: ilium
Insertion: femur
Action: abducts and medially rotates the thigh, used in walking and running

18 Gluteus minimus

Position: lateral area of buttocks, beneath gluteus medius
Origin: ilium
Insertion: femur
Action: abducts and rotates thigh, used in walking and running

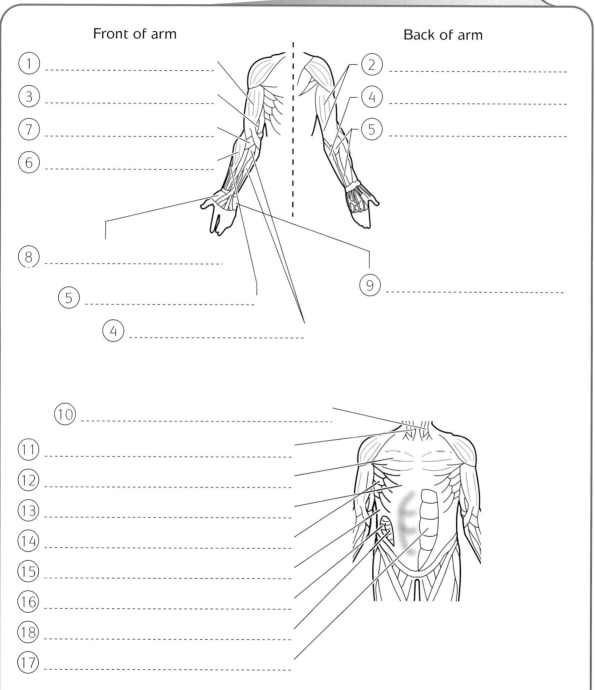

Front of arm

Back of arm

1
3
7
6

2
4
5

8

5

4

9

10
11
12
13
14
15
16
18
17

Figure 2.8 *Muscles of upper limbs and front of trunk and neck*

Label and colour the diagram in red using the information given on page 54.

Muscles of the upper limbs

1 Biceps brachii

Position: superficial muscle that runs down anterior surface of the humerus

Origin: scapula

Insertion: radius and flexor muscles in forearm

Action: flexes and supinates the forearm

2 Triceps

Position: superficial muscle found on posterior surface of humerus

Origin: humerus and scapula

Insertion: ulna

Action: extends the forearm

3 Brachialis

Position: found on the anterior aspect of humerus beneath the biceps

Origin: humerus

Insertion: ulna

Action: flexes the forearm

4 Flexors and 5 Extensors of the forearm

Position: forearm

Origin: flexors – humerus, radius and ulna; extensors – humerus

Insertion: flexors – carpals, metacarpals and phalanges; extensors – carpals, metacarpals and phalanges

Action: flexors flex the wrist and extensors extend the wrist

6 Brachioradialis

Position: superficial muscle found on the same side as the radius bone of forearm

Origin: humerus

Insertion: radius

Action: flexes, supinates and pronates forearm

7 Pronator teres

Position: anterior side of forearm, across elbow joint

Origin: humerus and ulna

Insertion: radius

Action: pronates and flexes forearm

8 **Thenar muscles**

Position: on the palm of the hand
Origin: carpals and metacarpals
Insertion: phalanx of the thumb
Action: the four thenar muscles act on the thumb. Movements include adduction, abduction and flexion of the thumb

9 **Hypothenar muscles**

Position: on the palm of the hand
Origin: carpals
Insertion: phalanx of little finger and the metacarpal near to little finger
Action: the three hypothenar muscles act on the little fingers. Movements include abduction and flexion of the little finger

> **Note**
>
> A single bone of the finger, thumb or toe is known as a phalanx.

Muscles of the anterior aspect of the trunk and neck

10 **Sternocleidomastoid**

Position: superficial muscle that runs from the top of the sternum to the clavicle and temporal bones
Origin: sternum and clavicle
Insertion: temporal bone
Action: both together, bends head forward. One muscle only rotates the head and draws it towards the opposite shoulder

11 **Platysma**

Position: superficial muscle that extends from the chin to the chest and covers the anterior of the neck
Origin: fascia over deltoid and pectoralis major muscles
Insertion: mandible
Action: depresses lower jaw and draws lower lip outwards and draws up the skin of the chest

12 **Pectoralis major**

Position: superficial muscle that covers the upper part of the chest
Origin: sternum, ribs and clavicle
Insertion: humerus
Action: adducts and medially rotates the arm

13 Pectoralis minor

Position:	small muscle found beneath pectoralis major
Origin:	ribs
Insertion:	scapula
Action:	draws shoulder downwards and also forwards

14 Serratus anterior

Position:	sides of ribcage below the armpits
Origin:	ribs
Insertion:	scapula
Action:	draws scapula forward as in pushing movements, such as used when boxing

Note

The linea alba is a tough, fibrous band that extends from the sternum to the pubis. In the later stages of pregnancy the linea alba stretches to increase the distance between the rectus abdominis muscles. It can be seen as a dark vertical line and is then known as the linea nigra.

15 External obliques

Position:	superficial muscles found laterally from side of waist to anterior of abdomen
Origin:	ribs
Insertion:	iliac crest and linea alba
Action:	twists trunk to opposite side

16 Internal obliques

Position:	found laterally on anterior of abdomen beneath external obliques
Origin:	iliac crest
Insertion:	ribs and linea alba
Action:	twists trunk to opposite side

17 Rectus abdominis

Position:	superficial muscles that extend the whole length of the abdomen. Medially the two muscles are attached to the linea alba
Origin:	pubic bone
Insertion:	sternum and lower ribs
Action:	supports abdominal organs and flexes vertebral column (as in bending forwards)

18 Transversus abdominis

Position: found laterally on front of abdomen, beneath internal oblique muscle
Origin: iliac crest, ribcage and vertebrae
Insertion: pubis, sternum and linea alba
Action: supports abdominal organs and flexes vertebral column

Task 2.8

Muscles of the lower limbs

Front of leg

3 ....
1d ....
2 ....
1b ....
1a ....
1c ....
10 ....
8 ....
11 ....

Back of leg

5a ....
5b ....
4 ....
5c ....
6 ....
7 ....
12 ....
9 ....

Plantar surface of foot

13 ....

14 ....

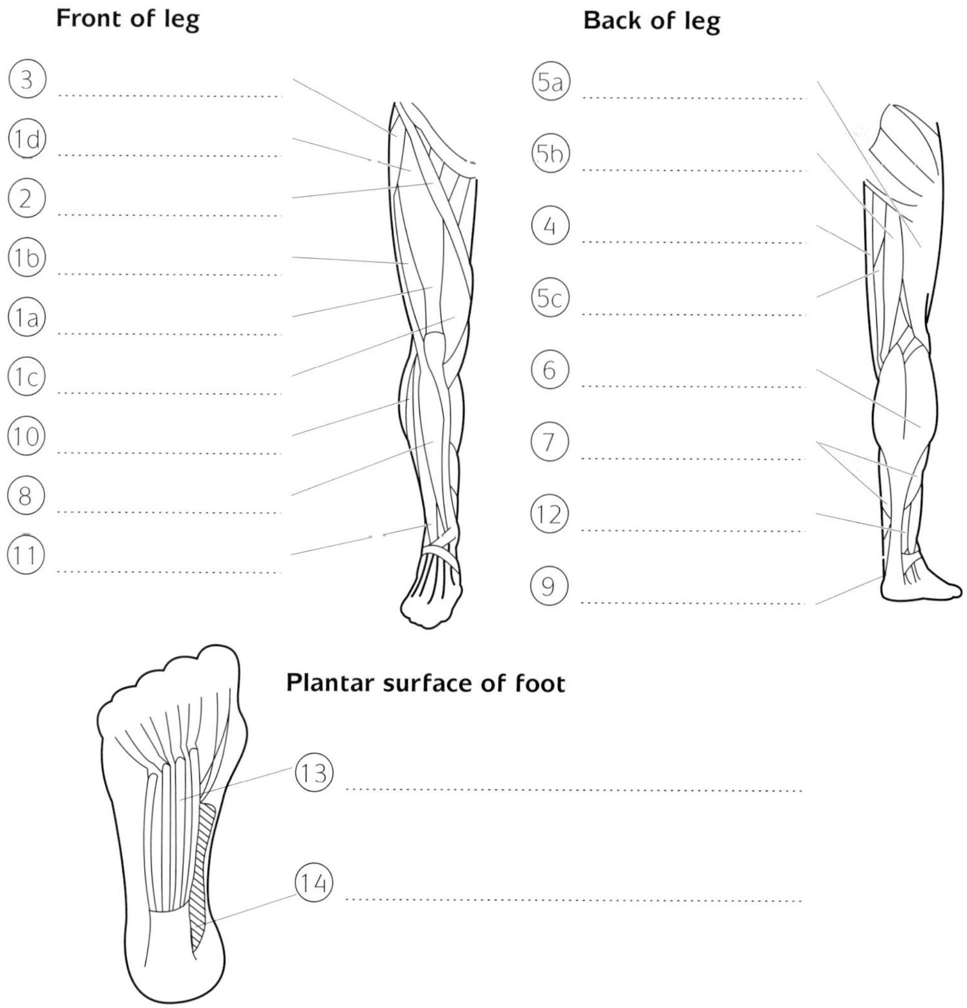

Figure 2.9 *Muscles of the lower limbs*

Label and lightly shade muscles with red pencil, using the information on page 58.

1 Quadriceps extensor

Position: group of four muscles located on the anterior of the thigh
        (a) rectus femoris
        (b) vastus lateralis
        (c) vastus medialis
        (d) vastus intermedius

Origin: ilium and femur

Insertion: patella and tibia

Action: extends (straightens) the leg and the rectus femoris, also flexes the thigh

2 Sartorius

Position: superficial muscle that crosses diagonally on anterior aspect of thigh

Origin: ilium

Insertion: tibia

Action: flexes (bends) knee and hip, and rotates the thigh laterally

3 Tensor fasciae latae

Position: superficial muscle found along lateral side of thigh

Origin: ilium

Insertion: tibia

Action: abducts and flexes the thigh

4 Adductors

Position: group of muscles found on medial aspect of thigh

Origin: pubis

Insertion: femur

Action: adduct the thigh

> **Note**
>
> A 'pulled groin' consists of tearing one or more of the adductor muscles or their tendons.

5 Hamstrings

Position: group of three muscles situated on the posterior of the thigh
        (a) biceps femoris
        (b) semitendinosus
        (c) semimembranosus

Origin: ischium

Insertion: tibia

Action: flexes the knee and extends the hip

6 Gastrocnemius

Position:	superficial muscle found at the back of lower leg
Origin:	femur
Insertion:	calcaneum bone (bone of the heel in the foot) via the Achilles tendon
Action:	plantar flexes the foot (draws foot downwards)

7 Soleus

Position:	at back of lower leg and is deep to gastrocnemius
Origin:	tibia and fibula
Insertion:	calcaneum bone via the Achilles tendon
Action:	plantar flexes foot

8 Tibialis anterior

Position:	superficial muscle situated down the shin bone
Origin:	tibia
Insertion:	tarsal and metatarsal bones
Action:	dorsiflexes (draws foot upwards)

9 Tibialis posterior

Position:	deepest muscle on back of lower leg
Origin:	tibia and fibula
Insertion:	tarsal and metatarsal bones
Action:	plantar flexes and inverts foot (draws foot inwards)

10 Flexor muscles – peroneus longus

Position:	down the outside of lower leg
Origin:	fibula
Insertion:	tarsal and first metatarsal bones
Action:	plantar flexes and everts foot (draws foot outwards). It supports the transverse and lateral longitudinal arches of the feet

11 Extensors hallucis longus

Position:	down front of lower leg
Origin:	fibula
Insertion:	phalanx of big toe
Action:	extends the big toe

12 Flexor hallucis longus

Position:	outer side and towards the back of lower leg
Origin:	fibula
Insertion:	phalanx of big toe

Action: flexes the big toe, inverts and plantar flexes foot. Also supports medial longitudinal arch of foot

13 Flexor digitorum brevis

Position: plantar surface of foot
Origin: calcaneus (bone of heel of foot)
Insertion: phalanges of toes, except big toe
Action: flexes all toes, except big toe

14 Abductor hallucis

Position: plantar surface of foot
Origin: calcaneus (bone of heel of foot)
Insertion: phalanx of big toe
Action: abducts and flexes big toe

Task 2.9

To help you remember the names of the muscles, make copies of the muscle tables and then highlight the different groups, eg blue for muscle, green for position, orange for action, and so on. Cut up your table copies. Mix the name, origin, insertion, position and action all up and try to match them back together.

Effects of massage on the muscular system

◆ The blood supply to the muscle will be increased during massage, bringing fresh oxygen and nutrients and removing waste products such as lactic acid, so this can help to alleviate muscle fatigue.

- Massage will help to relieve pain, stiffness and fatigue in muscles as the waste products are removed and normal functioning is quickly restored. The increased oxygen and nutrients will aid tissue repair and recovery of the muscle.

- Massage can help the breakdown of fibrositic nodules, also termed knots, that develop within a muscle due to tension, injuries or poor posture. They are commonly found in the shoulder area.

- Massage helps to increase the tone of the muscles and delay wasting away of muscles through lack of use.

- The muscles are warmed due to the increased blood flow. Warm muscles contract more efficiently than cold muscles, and so massage prior to exercise will help reduce the incidence of injury.

- Massage will help to relax muscles that are tense and contracted.

- Massage will help to reduce adhesions (i.e. scar tissue) in muscle, which may have been caused by an injury.

CARDIOVASCULAR SYSTEM

The cardiovascular system consists of the heart, blood and blood vessels. The function of the heart is to act as a pump to move the blood around the body. The blood carries oxygen and nutrients, and is transported in the body in a series of pipes called blood vessels.

Pulmonary and general circulation

The pulmonary circulation is the circulation of blood between the heart and the lungs. The general circulation is the circulation of blood from the left side of the heart to the rest of the body's tissues.

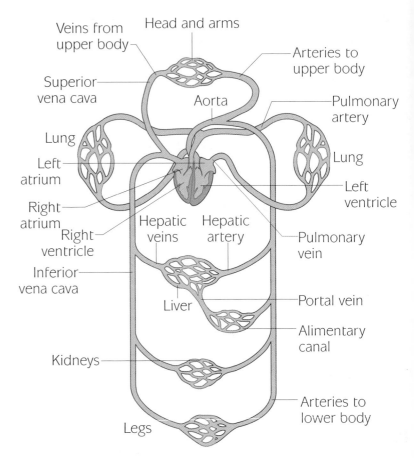

Figure 2.10 *Pulmonary and general circulatory systems*

Blood

Plasma is the liquid part of the blood and mainly consists of water. Many substances can travel in the blood plasma, including blood cells, hormones, nutrients and the waste products produced by cells.

Functions of the blood

The functions of the blood include:

◆ clotting of the blood to prevent excess blood loss if an injury should occur to the body

◆ attacking of harmful organisms such as bacteria. The white blood cells protect the body against disease

◆ removal of carbon dioxide and waste from the cells

♦ delivery of oxygen, nutrients and hormones to the cells of the body. Heat is also transported around the body from the muscles and liver, which helps regulate the body temperature.

Red blood cells

The function of red blood cells is to carry oxygen around the body and deliver it to the cells. The cells use the oxygen and nutrients and produce carbon dioxide as a result. Carbon dioxide can be carried away by the red blood cells and taken back to the lungs to be breathed out.

White blood cells

White blood cells help protect the body from disease. They are called phagocytes, which means they are able to engulf and digest (eat) bacteria and any other harmful matter. Most of them are able to change their shape so can squeeze through small spaces, and are therefore able to reach almost anywhere in the body.

Platelets

Platelets are involved with the clotting process of the blood following an injury to the body. Their function is to help prevent the loss of blood from damaged blood vessels by forming a plug.

Blood vessels

Blood is transported around the body in blood vessels. These blood vessels are called arteries, arterioles, capillaries, venules and veins, and form an intricate network within the body.

Arteries

Arteries have thick, elastic, muscular walls because the blood within them is carried under high pressure, due to the pumping action of the heart. They carry blood away from the heart. Most arteries carry oxygenated blood, with the exception of the pulmonary arteries, which carry deoxygenated blood away from the heart to the lungs. Arteries are generally deep seated, except where they cross on a pulse spot, such as radial artery in the wrist and carotid artery in the neck where a pulse can be felt. As arteries get further from the heart they branch off and become smaller. The oxygenated blood eventually reaches very small arteries called arterioles.

Capillaries

Arterioles are connected to the capillaries. Capillaries are the smallest vessels, about a hundredth of a millimetre thick. Unlike arteries and veins, the walls of the capillaries are thin enough to allow certain substances to pass through them, in a process known as capillary exchange. Oxygen and nutrients are delivered to the cells of the body, and carbon dioxide and waste products are removed.

The capillaries connect with larger vessels called venules. Now that oxygen has been removed from the blood and given to cells, and carbon dioxide has been picked up from the cells, by the time the blood reaches the venules it has become deoxygenated.

Note

There are over 60,000 miles of blood vessels in the human body.

Veins

Blood flows through the venules until it reaches larger vessels called veins. The veins carry blood, called venous blood, towards the direction of the heart. Their walls are thinner and less elastic than arteries. Veins carry deoxygenated blood, with the exception of the pulmonary veins. Pulmonary veins carry oxygenated blood from the lungs towards the heart. Veins are nearer the surface of the body than the arteries. Unlike the other blood vessels, veins contain valves, which prevent the blood from flowing backwards. Examples of veins include the internal jugular veins that carry blood away from the head and neck, and the external jugular that carries blood away from the scalp, and both are found in the neck.

Unlike arteries, the veins carry blood at low pressure because the blood flow is not helped by the pumping action of the heart. Blood in the veins is moved through the body by the squeezing action of the voluntary muscles, such as during walking, and the involuntary muscles, such as the movement of breathing. Therefore, exercise and massage are particularly useful to help the venous flow.

Task 2.10

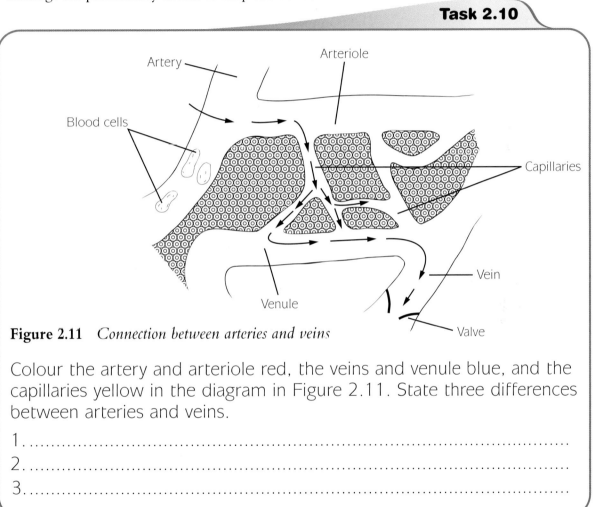

Figure 2.11 *Connection between arteries and veins*

Colour the artery and arteriole red, the veins and venule blue, and the capillaries yellow in the diagram in Figure 2.11. State three differences between arteries and veins.

1. ....
2. ....
3. ....

Blood shunting

There are points along blood vessels where the small arteries have direct contact with veins. They are called shunt vessels and allow blood to pass from an artery directly to a vein, so it does not enter the capillaries. Blood shunting occurs, for instance, after eating a heavy meal; the blood is directed to the intestines to help digest food. It is therefore not advised to have a treatment after a big meal as the massage will cause the blood flow to be diverted to the skin and muscles.

Pulse

The pumping action of the heart is so strong it can be felt as a pulse in the arteries, especially those that lie close to the surface of the body, such as the radial artery in the wrist and the carotid artery in the neck. The number of pulse beats per minute represent the heart rate. The average pulse of an adult is between 60 and 80 beats per minute. Factors that increase the pulse rate include exercise, drugs and emotion.

Blood pressure

When blood reaches the capillaries it is vital that oxygen and nutrients pass out of the blood and into the cells. It is the pressure of blood that forces fluid out through the capillary walls. Therefore, it is important for the body to maintain the correct level of blood pressure.

With each heartbeat the heart contracts and the blood pressure inside it will increase. Blood pressure measures the force with which the heart pumps blood around the body. It is the force of pressure the blood exerts against the walls of the arteries. Blood pressure can be likened to the pressure in a hosepipe, which increases and decreases as the tap is turned on and off.

A normal blood pressure will measure around 120 mmHg systolic and 80 mmHg diastolic, or 120/80. A raised blood pressure may be due to damaged blood vessels that are less elastic or have a partial blockage, and a weak heart will show low blood pressure. People who exercise regularly often have slightly lower than normal blood pressure. Exercise helps to strengthen the heart, so it has to do less work to pump the same amount of blood.

Effect of massage on the cardiovascular system

♦ Massage causes the blood vessels to compress, forcing blood forwards; as pressure is released the blood vessels return to normal size and blood rushes in to fill the space created. Reddening of the skin called **erythema** results. Fresh, oxygenated blood and nutrients are brought to the area and so will nourish the tissues and help with tissue repair. Waste products (metabolic waste) are removed and carried away by the veins. A build up of waste products can cause pain and stiffness and so massage can help to relieve these symptoms.

♦ Massage movements such as effleurage (stroking) will help to speed the flow of blood in the veins back to the heart: **venous return**. This is why strokes are performed in the direction of the venous flow.

♦ The flow of blood through the veins is speeded up by regular leg massage treatment. The massage helps to stop overloading of the veins, therefore helping to prevent varicose veins.

♦ Regular relaxing massages may help to reduce high blood pressure.

♦ Massage causes the superficial capillaries in the skin to dilate, producing erythema.

LYMPHATIC SYSTEM

Have you noticed how certain glands swell up when you are ill, such as the glands in the neck, which inflame during a throat infection? The glands you can feel are lymph nodes. Lymph nodes, lymph, lymph vessels and lymphatic ducts all make up the lymphatic system, which is closely related to the blood circulation.

The functions of the lymphatic system

The three main functions of the lymphatic system are:

1   to help the body to fight infection

2   to distribute fluid in the body. Lymphatic vessels drain approximately 3 litres of excess tissue fluid daily from tissue spaces

3   to enable the transport of fats. Fats are passed from the small intestine into lymphatic vessels and eventually into the bloodstream.

How is lymph derived?

Blood does not flow into the tissues but remains inside the blood vessels. However, plasma from the blood is able to seep through the capillary walls and enter the spaces between the tissues. This fluid provides the cells with nutrients and oxygen. It has now become tissue fluid. More fluid passes out of the blood capillaries than is returned. The excess tissue fluid passes into the lymphatic capillaries and now becomes lymph. Lymph is similar to blood plasma but contains more white blood cells.

Lymph is a watery, colourless fluid that passes through the lymph nodes. Lymph nodes filter out harmful substances from the lymph, such as bacteria, which could cause an infection in the body. They contain specialised white blood cells that destroy harmful substances by ingesting them and also produce antibodies, which stop the growth of bacteria and their harmful action. During an infection there are more bacteria and so the lymph nodes produce more lymphocytes to destroy them. This causes the lymph nodes to enlarge and is a sign that the glands are working to fight the infection.

Lymph vessels

Lymph travels towards the direction of the heart and is carried in vessels, which begin as lymphatic capillaries. Lymph capillaries are blind-ended tubes, situated between cells, and are found throughout the body. The lymphatic capillaries allow tissue fluid to pass into them but not out due to the structure of their walls.

Lymphatic capillaries join up and become wider tubes, known as lymphatic vessels. The lymph vessels generally run parallel to the veins. These vessels are similar to veins as they contain valves, although they generally have thinner walls. The lymph flows around the body through these lymph vessels and will pass through a number of lymph nodes to be filtered. Eventually the lymph will be passed into lymphatic ducts.

Lymph nodes

There are approximately 600 bean-shaped lymph nodes scattered throughout the body. They lie mainly in groups around the groin, breast and armpits and around the major blood vessels of the abdomen and chest.

Important groups of lymph nodes in the head and neck are occipital (1), submandibular (2), deep cervical (3) and superficial cervical glands (4). Important groups of lymph nodes of the rest of the body include axillary (5), abdominal (6), inguinal (7), popliteal (8) and supratrochlear nodes (9) (see task 2.11).

Lymphatic ducts

The lymphatic ducts are known as the thoracic duct (10) and right lymphatic duct (11). Lymph from the lower body and upper left side of the body passes into the thoracic duct. The thoracic duct drains the lymph directly into the left subclavian vein, so that it is returned to the blood circulation.

The right lymphatic duct drains lymph from the upper right-hand side of the body. The lymph passes into the right subclavian vein where it will join the venous blood to become part of the blood circulation once again.

Task 2.11

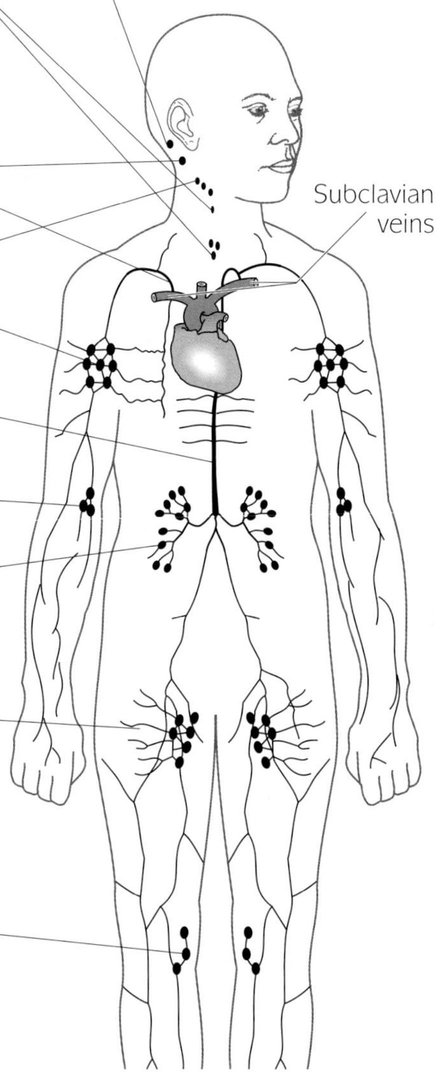
1
3
11
4
5
2
10
9
6
7
8
Subclavian veins

Use yellow shading to colour the lymph glands and lymphatic vessels. Colour the thoracic and right lymphatic duct green. Use red to colour the subclavian veins and heart. Use the information on page 69 to label the diagram.

Figure 2.12 *The glands of the neck and body*

The lymphatic system does not have a pump like the heart, but like veins relies on the movement of the body and the contraction of the skeletal muscles. The squeezing action of the muscles will force the lymph along its vessels. Involuntary actions such as breathing and the heart beating will also help the movement of lymph through the vessels.

Note

Excess fluid that accumulates in the tissues causing swelling is known as oedema or fluid retention. It is commonly seen around the ankles. It often occurs in women just before a period, due to a hormone imbalance. Exercise and massage are both beneficial for this condition. However, it can sometimes be a sign of a more serious disease, such as kidney disease, especially if generalised. The therapist would need to ensure it was a non-medical oedema before giving a massage treatment.

Effects of massage on the lymphatic system

◆ Massage speeds up the flow of lymph in lymph vessels.

◆ Massage can help reduce or even prevent oedema (fluid retention).

NERVOUS SYSTEM

Note

The nervous system consists of the brain, spinal cord, nerves and sense organs. It controls all the bodily systems and provides the most rapid means of communication in the body. The nervous system can be likened to a telephone network with messages continually being passed through wires. In the body the messages are in the form of electrical impulses, which pass from neurone (nerve cell) to neurone. There are billions of neurones within the body and their function is to transmit nerve impulses.

The fastest nerve signals can travel at 250 mph.

Nerves

A large number of neurones are arranged in bundles and form nerves. Unlike other cells neurones cannot divide and reproduce themselves.

Divisions of the nervous system

The nervous system can be divided into the central, peripheral and autonomic nervous system.

Central nervous system (CNS)

The central nervous system consists of the brain and spinal cord. The brain is the most important part of the system and contains 100 billion neurones. The brain receives and stores messages as well as transmitting them to all parts of the body to stimulate organs to do their work.

Spinal cord

The spinal cord extends downwards through the vertebral column ending level at the lumbar vertebrae. It contains about 100 million neurones. The function of the spinal cord is to provide communication between the brain and all parts of the body.

The cerebrospinal fluid (CSF) is similar to blood plasma in composition. It protects the brain and spinal cord by acting as a cushion and shock absorber.

Peripheral nervous system

This system is concerned with all nerves situated outside the central nervous system, including motor and sensory nerves.

Motor nerves carry nerve impulses from the brain, through the spinal cord to the skeletal muscles, glands and smooth muscular tissue to stimulate them into carrying out their work.

Sensory nerves carry nerve impulses from sensory nerve endings in organs such as the skin, and transmit the impulse to the brain and spinal cord.

There are 31 pairs of spinal nerves that originate from the spinal cord, and emerge between the vertebrae. The nerves are either sensory, motor or mixed (containing both types). The spinal nerves are named according to the region of the spinal cord from which they emerge.

Task 2.12

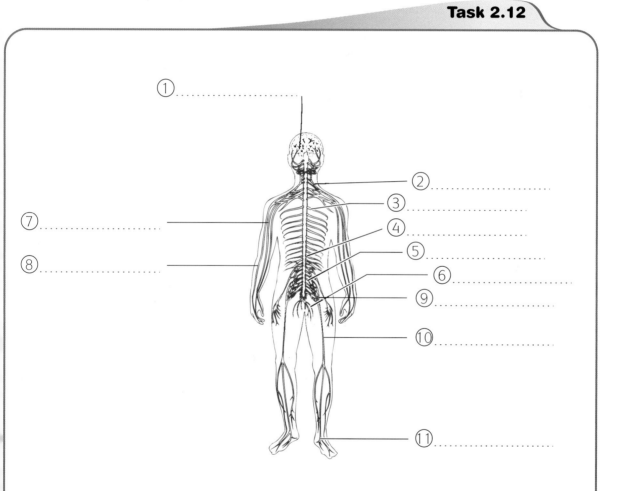

Figure 2.13 *The nerves of the body*

Label the diagram, matching the numbers to the numbered terms in the following text. Use yellow shading to colour the nerves and brown for the brain and spinal cord.

1	Cranial nerves	5	Sacral nerves	9	Femoral nerve
2	Cervical nerves	6	Coccygeal nerves	10	Sciatic nerve
3	Thoracic nerves	7	Median nerve	11	Tibial nerve
4	Lumbar nerves	8	Radial nerve		

Note

The sciatic nerves are the longest nerves of the body and arise from the sacral plexus. They run down the back of each leg from pelvis to the knees, and give branches to the lower legs and feet. They carry messages to and from all parts of the leg.

Autonomic nervous system

The autonomic nervous system has two parts called the sympathetic and parasympathetic, which have opposite effects. Each organ has a sympathetic and parasympathetic nerve supply.

The sympathetic nerves are responsible for actions in time of stress. In an emergency, such as when feeling threatened, the sympathetic nervous system has immediate effects on the body. Sympathetic nerves stimulate the adrenal glands to produce the hormone adrenalin. The hormone is distributed quickly by the blood and stimulates organs into greater activity. When the emergency is over the parasympathetic system will return the body to its normal state.

The parasympathetic nerves control everyday bodily activities such as digestion and urination. It is directed towards relaxation and restorative processes. The heart rate slows, blood pressure drops and the digestive system becomes active.

Effects of massage on the nervous system

◆ A relaxing slow massage, using lots of effleurage, produces a soothing, sedative effect on the nerve endings.

◆ An invigorating massage using tapotement movements will have a stimulating effect on the nerves and body.

◆ An increased blood flow helps to provide nutrients for nerve cells.

ENDOCRINE SYSTEM

Task 2.13

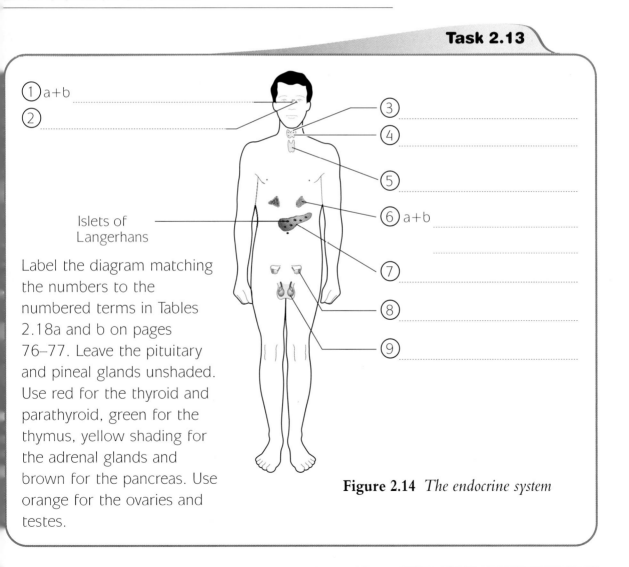

① a+b

②

③

④

⑤

⑥ a+b

⑦

⑧

⑨

Islets of Langerhans

Label the diagram matching the numbers to the numbered terms in Tables 2.18a and b on pages 76–77. Leave the pituitary and pineal glands unshaded. Use red for the thyroid and parathyroid, green for the thymus, yellow shading for the adrenal glands and brown for the pancreas. Use orange for the ovaries and testes.

Figure 2.14 *The endocrine system*

Table 2.18a The endocrine glands – pituitary gland

Endocrine gland	Hormone released	Target organ or organs affected by hormone	What does hormone control or stimulate production of?
1a Anterior pituitary	ACTH – adrenocorticotrophic hormone	Adrenal glands	Controls activity of adrenal cortex
	TSH – thyroid stimulating hormone	Thyroid gland	Controls activity of thyroid gland
	Growth hormone	All organs	Controls growth of skeleton, muscles and organs
	Prolactin	Breasts	Stimulates milk production
	FSH – follicle stimulating hormone	Ovaries and testes	Stimulates the development of eggs and production of oestrogen in females. In males stimulates sperm production
	LH – leutinising hormone	Ovaries and testes	Stimulates egg release from ovaries and production of progesterone. In males stimulates the testes to make testosterone
1b Posterior pituitary	Anti-diuretic hormone	Kidneys	Controls water balance in the body
	Oxytocin	Breasts	Releases milk from breasts during suckling

Table 2.18b Endocrine glands relating to the rest of the body

Endocrine gland	Hormone released	Action of hormone
2 Pineal	Melatonin	Helps to control body rhythms such as sleeping and waking patterns
3 Thyroid	Thyroxine	Controls the metabolism
4 Parathyroid	Parathormone	Controls calcium levels in the blood
5 Thymus	Thymosin	Involved with the production of lymphocytes
6a Adrenal cortex	Sex corticoids	Controls changes in males and females during puberty
	Glucocorticoids	Helps regulate nutrient levels in the blood
	Mineral corticoids	Helps maintain balance of minerals in body
6b Adrenal medulla	Adrenalin and noradrenalin	Prepares body for fight or flight response
7 Pancreas	Insulin and glucagon	Controls sugar levels in the blood
8 Ovaries	Oestrogen and progesterone	Controls female secondary sexual characteristics such as breasts, curves and pubic hair
9. Testes	Testosterone	Controls male secondary sexual characteristics such as bodily hair, deep voice and muscular development

Effects of massage on the endocrine system

◆ When the body is under stress, certain hormones are stimulated, especially from the adrenal glands. Massage can reduce the amount of stress hormones released as it helps to reduce stress and promote relaxation in the body.

◆ Can help to regulate periods, if the menstrual cycle is disturbed due to the effects of stress.

RESPIRATORY SYSTEM

Every living cell in the body needs oxygen. We obtain the oxygen we require from the air that we breathe. Inspiration is the movement of air into the lungs and expiration is the movement of air out of the lungs. The respiratory system is concerned with the exchange of gases between the lungs and the blood and consists of a number of organs.

Task 2.14

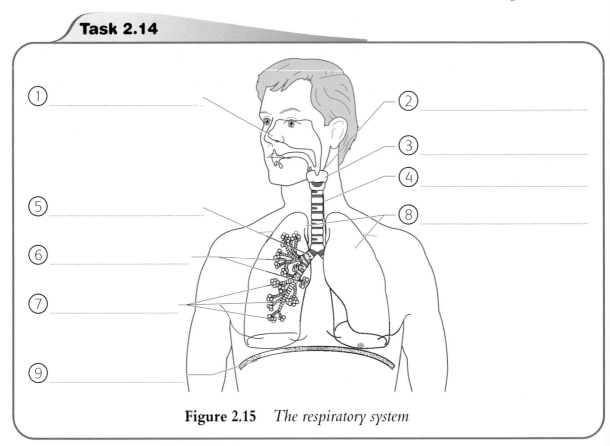

Figure 2.15 *The respiratory system*

Label the diagram, matching the numbers to the numbered terms in Table 2.19 below. Shade the following using a red pencil: nose, sinuses, pharynx, larynx, trachea, bronchi and bronchioles. Use yellow to colour the alveoli and diaphragm. Use brown for the lungs.

Organs of the respiratory system

Table 2.19 The structure of the respiratory organs

Structure	Description
1 Nose	Air is breathed in through the nose and becomes moistened and warmed. Coarse hairs filter out large dust particles.
2 Pharynx (throat)	The pharynx is a tube and allows air to enter the larynx.
3 Larynx	The larynx is the voice box and is a short passageway linking the pharynx to the trachea.
4 Trachea (windpipe)	The trachea or windpipe is a tube and acts as a passageway for air. The trachea extends into the thorax (chest cavity) and branches off to form the bronchi. Tiny, hair-like cilia trap dust and harmful substances and carry them towards the throat. (Nicotine paralyses cilia so smokers cough to remove foreign particles from the lungs instead.)
5 Bronchi	The bronchi are two tubes, individually known as a bronchus, which carry air into the lungs.
6 Bronchioles	The bronchi divide into branches called bronchioles. The bronchioles become progressively smaller until they join on to the alveoli.
7 Alveoli	The round sac-like shape of the alveoli ensures a large surface area for exchange of gases. The alveoli have very thin walls and each alveolus is surrounded by a network of capillaries; this ensures that an efficient exchange of oxygen and carbon dioxide can take place.
8 Lungs	The lungs are large organs situated at either side of the thoracic cavity and are separated by the heart.
9 Diaphragm	The diaphragm is a large, dome-shaped muscle found directly under the lungs. It separates the thoracic cavity from the abdominal cavity.

Gas exchange in the lungs

Air is breathed into the lungs where oxygen diffuses through the walls of the alveoli and passes into the blood. It is picked up by the red blood cells and taken around the body to provide oxygen for the body's cells. The cells produce carbon dioxide, which has to be removed from the body. The carbon dioxide diffuses from the cells into the surrounding capillaries. When it reaches the capillaries surrounding the alveoli, it passes through the alveoli walls where it will be breathed out. The deoxygenated blood becomes oxygenated once again. This is a process that is continually happening and is essential for life.

The mechanism of breathing

During inspiration (breathing in) the intercostal muscles found between the ribs contract, moving the ribs up and out. The diaphragm muscle also contracts and so the dome shape is flattened. This increases the space in the lungs and causes air to be automatically drawn into them. This process can be likened to having your hands glued to a balloon (which represents the lung attached to the chest wall) and pulling it wider to increase the space inside.

During expiration (breathing out) the intercostal muscles relax and the ribs return to their resting position. The diaphragm relaxes, returning to its original dome shape. This causes the space in the lungs to get smaller, thus forcing air out of them.

Effects of massage on the respiratory system

- Massage to the chest muscles will help relax the chest and so breathing may be improved, especially if the client suffers from tightness in the chest often associated with anxiety problems.

- Massage will increase the blood circulation to the lung tissue helping to bring nutrients and rid the body of carbon dioxide. This will improve the condition of the lungs.

DIGESTIVE SYSTEM

The digestive system changes the food we eat into small, simple substances that can be absorbed into the bloodstream and used by the body to produce energy or as building materials for repairing itself or growing.

Food contains substances called nutrients found within five basic food groups: protein, carbohydrates, fats, vitamins and minerals. Although fibre is not nutritionally valuable it is important for a healthy diet. All foods contain some nutrients, but hardly any food contains them all. For the body to remain healthy a variety of foods needs to be eaten.

Table 2.20 The food groups

Food group	Function	Good sources
Protein	Vital for growth and repair of cells	Meat, fish, eggs, milk, cheese
Carbohydrates	Provide energy for the body	Potatoes, bread, sugar, cereals, pasta
Fats	Provide energy for the body	Butter, lard, vegetable oil, cheese
Vitamins/minerals	Essential for growth and general health	Fruit and vegetables
Fibre	Helps keep muscles of the intestines exercised and provides bulk to satisfy appetite. Prevents constipation	Vegetables, fruit, cereals and wholemeal foods

The digestive tract, also known as the alimentary canal, is more than 10 metres long and begins at the mouth and ends at the anus. Food takes on average 24 hours to pass through the digestive tract.

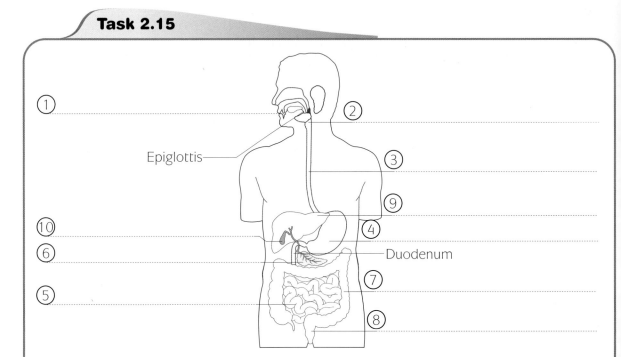

① ② ③ ⑨ ⑩ ⑥ ⑤ ④ ⑦ ⑧

Epiglottis

Duodenum

Figure 2.16 *The organs of the digestive system*

Label the diagram, matching the numbers to the numbered terms in Table 2.21 opposite. Use pink shading for the mouth, oesophagus, stomach, small intestine, large intestine and rectum. Use brown for the liver, green for the gall bladder and yellow for the pancreas.

Table 2.21 Structure of the digestive system

Structure	Description
1 Mouth	The teeth help break down the food during chewing. There are three main pairs of salivary glands, which produce saliva. The saliva lubricates the food and in most people contains an enzyme called salivary amylase. This enzyme begins the breakdown of starch in cooked foods. Starch is found in foods like bread, potatoes and grains.
2 Pharynx	The muscles of the pharynx (throat) push the food down into the oesophagus (food pipe). A flap of cartilage known as the epiglottis prevents the food being swallowed from entering into the lungs.
3 Oesophagus	This is the foodpipe, a muscular tube leading to the stomach. Waves of contractions (peristalsis) occur in the muscles of the oesophagus wall. The walls squeeze and relax to push food along the digestive tract.
4 Stomach	This is a muscular, J-shaped bag-like organ situated on the left side of the abdominal cavity beneath the diaphragm.
5 Small intestine	The food passes into the small intestine, which is over 6 metres long and is the place where most of the nutrients are absorbed.
6 Pancreas	The pancreas is a gland situated behind the stomach and is about 15 cm long. It produces enzymes, which are substances that help break down the food.
7 Large intestine	The large intestine, also called the colon, is about 1.5 metres long and is divided into the ascending, transverse and descending colon. Any remaining undigested food and fibre (roughage) is now waste matter and passes from the small intestine into the large intestine in liquid form. Any remaining nutrients and water are removed from this waste matter and reabsorbed into the body. This results in solid faeces being formed.
8 Rectum	The rectum is about 13 cm long and has two sphincter muscles, known as the anus, through which waste matter is expelled.
9 Liver	The liver is a large organ found in the upper right corner of the abdomen and extends across to the left side. It lies below the diaphragm and is mostly protected by the ribs. Its functions include storing and filtering blood, secreting bile, detoxification of substances, e.g. alcohol, storage of vitamins A, D, E and K, and iron, and storage of glycogen, which can be broken down into glucose and used for energy by the body when required.
10 Gall bladder	The gall bladder stores bile, a greenish fluid produced by the liver. After food has been eaten bile is released and travels to the duodenum where it begins to break down fats.

Effects of massage on the digestive system

◆ Massage on the abdomen helps to stimulate peristalsis and promote the movement of waste matter through the colon.

◆ Abdominal massage helps to relieve flatulence and constipation.

◆ Massage over the abdomen can help to soothe the nerves of the alimentary canal, so can help relieve intestinal spasm, associated with conditions such as irritable bowel syndrome.

REPRODUCTIVE SYSTEMS

The reproductive systems of males and females ensure new human life can be created. This can only happen when a women's ovum (egg) is fertilised by a man's sperm.

The female reproductive organs are situated within the pelvic cavity and the pelvic bones help to protect them. The pelvic cavity is wider in the female than the male to allow more space for childbirth.

Male reproductive system

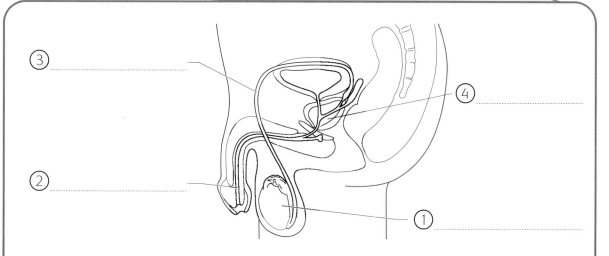

Figure 2.17 *The male reproductive system*

Label the diagram, matching the numbers to the numbered terms in Table 2.22 below. Use red shading to colour the testes and brown for the prostate gland. Shade the urethra and vas deferens yellow. Use pink for the penis.

Table 2.22 Structure of the male reproductive system

Structure	Description
1 Testes	Two oval glands that produce sperm and testosterone.
2 Urethra	Acts as a passageway for semen and urine.
3 Vas deferens	About 45 cm long and passes from testes to urethra. Acts as passageway for sperm.
4 Prostate gland	About the size of a chestnut and lies under the bladder. It surrounds the beginning of the urethra. Secretes milky fluid that makes up 25% of semen.

Female reproductive system

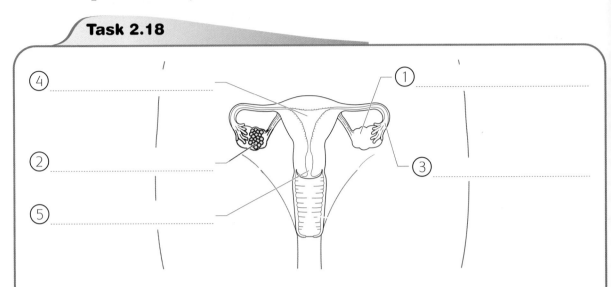

Figure 2.18 *The female reproductive system*

Label the diagram, matching the numbers to the numbered terms in Table 2.23 below. Use yellow shading for the ovaries and ova. Use brown shading for the fallopian tubes, uterus and cervix, and red for the vagina.

Table 2.23 Structure of the female reproductive system

Structure	Description
1 Ovaries	Glands about 3 cm long each, found either side of uterus. Release hormones oestrogen and progesterone.
2 Ova (eggs)	Egg produced by ovaries and released into fallopian tube.
3 Fallopian tubes	Act as passageway for sperms to reach the ovum (egg) and is where ovum becomes fertilised.
4 Uterus (womb)	Located at centre of pelvic cavity, the bladder in front and the rectum behind. Fertilised ovum will attach itself to the lining of the uterus and grow to become a baby.
5 Cervix	Short, narrow passageway found at bottom end of uterus. Dilates during childbirth. It opens into the vagina.

Breasts

The function of breasts is to produce milk (lactation) after childbirth. They lie over the pectoralis major and serratus anterior muscles and have a vast network of blood and lymphatic vessels. They consist mainly of glandular and fatty (adipose) tissue.

Task 2.18

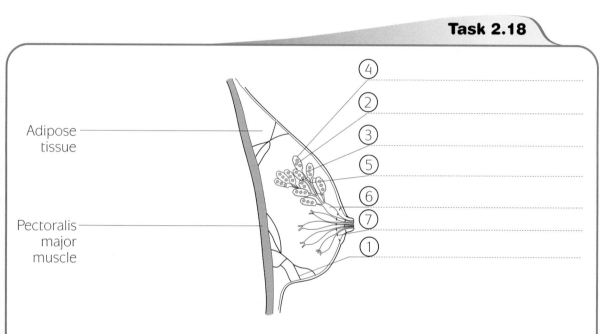

Adipose tissue

Pectoralis major muscle

Figure 2.19 *The structures of the breast*

Label the diagram, matching the numbers to the numbered terms in Table 2.24 on page 88. Colour the diagram using yellow for the lobes, lobules, alveoli, milk ducts and lactiferous sinuses. Use red to colour the Cooper's ligaments, areola and nipple.

Table 2.24 The structures of the breast

Structure	Decription
1 Cooper's ligaments	Made up of strands of connective tissue and help to support breasts. Become slack with age or prolonged strain such as vigorous exercise causing the breasts to sag.
2 Lobes	Breast contains about 20 lobes.
3 Lobules	Each lobe contains several lobules. Lobules contain glands called alveoli.
4 Alveoli	Milk is produced in the alveoli glands and passes into the milk ducts.
5 Milk ducts	Carries milk to lactiferous sinuses.
6 Lactiferous sinuses	Act as storage for milk. The milk then passes into ducts to be released by nipple.
7 Areola	Pigmented area that surrounds the nipple.

Lymphatic drainage of the breasts

The lymphatic drainage of the breast is extensive and drains mostly into the axillary lymph vessels and nodes under the armpits. If breast cancer develops this extensive lymph drainage allows the spread of cancer elsewhere in the body.

Effects of massage on the reproductive system

◆ The increased blood flow will help bring oxygen and nutrients to the area and remove waste products, therefore improving the health of organs of the reproductive systems.

◆ Although generally we do not work directly on the breasts, massage around the breast area will help to improve lymph drainage and so reduce fluid retention, common around the time of menstruation.

URINARY SYSTEM

The urinary system filters the blood and produces urine to ensure the body gets rid of unwanted substances that could be harmful. It consists of two kidneys, two ureters, bladder and the urethra.

Task 2.19

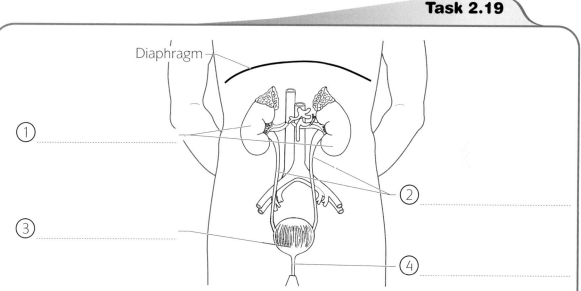

Figure 2.20 *The urinary system*

I abel the diagram, matching the numbers to the numbered terms in the text below. Use brown shading for the kidneys and ureters, and yellow for the bladder and urethra. Use red for the arteries and blue for the veins.

1 Kidneys

The kidneys are two bean-shaped organs. Each would almost cover the area of a woman's hand and is about 2 centimetres thick. They are positioned in the lower back just above the waist, are mostly protected by the ribs and are surrounded by a thick layer of fat.

Note

The right kidney is slightly lower than the left because of the large space occupied by the liver.

An important function of the kidneys is to filter the blood, in other words to clean it and get rid of any unwanted substances (waste). Many of these substances are toxic and would result in death if allowed to accumulate in the body.

The kidneys help to control this balance by removing water from the blood vessels that enter them and by producing urine. They do this without affecting the other important substances in the blood.

2 Ureters

Urine is formed in the kidneys and consists of 95 per cent water, 2 per cent mineral salts and 3 per cent waste products. It passes from the kidneys into two tubes called the ureters. The ureters are about 30 centimetres long and join on to the back of the bladder.

3 Bladder

Urine is stored in a muscular sac called the bladder. When a sufficient amount of urine is collected in the bladder, the desire to urinate (micturate) will be produced.

Note

Cystitis is an infection of the bladder lining, often caused by a bacterial infection. Cystitis is more common in women than men because of the shortness of the woman's urethra.

4 Urethra

The urethra is a narrow tube leading from the bladder to outside the body and is shorter in females than males. It acts as a passageway for urine and for sperm in males.

Massage

Although the kidneys are mostly protected by the ribs and muscles and are deeply embedded in fat they are delicate organs so care has to be taken when massaging so as not to apply too much pressure.

Effects of massage on the urinary system

◆ The increased lymphatic flow may cause an increased amount of urine to pass to the bladder.

Task 2.20

Research the effects that massage has on the various systems and complete Table 2.25 below.

Table 2.25 The effects of massage on the bodily systems

Bodily system	One effect massage has on this system
Skin	
Skeletal/joints	
Muscular	
Cardiovascular	
Lymphatic	
Nervous	
Endocrine	
Respiratory	
Digestive	
Reproductive	
Urinary	

1. Give **3** examples of different types of cells found in the body.

    . . . .

2. List the **5** layers of the epidermis.

    . . . .

    . . . .

    . . . .

3. Name the layers found below the epidermis.

    . . . .

    . . . .

    . . . .

4. Name and describe **3** structures found in the skin.

    . . . .

    . . . .

    . . . .

5. List **3** functions of the skin.

    . . . .

    . . . .

    . . . .

    . . . .

    . . . .

6. List **5** infectious skin diseases.

. . . .

. . . .

. . . .

7. Give **5** examples of skin conditions that are not infectious.

. . . .

. . . .

. . . .

8. State **3** functions of the skeleton.

. . . .

. . . .

. . . .

9. What are ligaments and tendons?

. . . .

. . . .

. . . .

10. Name the **3** main types of joints found in the body and give an example of each.

. . . .

. . . .

. . . .

11. List the **3** types of muscles found in the body and give an example of each.

. . . .

. . . .

. . . .

12. Briefly describe 'muscle fatigue'.

. . . .

. . . .

. . . .

. . . .

. . . .

13. What is cramp and how can gentle massage help this condition?

. . . .

. . . .

. . . .

14. State **2** functions of the blood.

. . . .

. . . .

. . . .

15. Draw a diagram showing how arteries, capillaries and veins link together.

16. Give a description of blood pressure.

. . . .

. . . .

. . . .

17. What is erythema?

. . . .

. . . .

. . . .

18. State **3** functions of the lymphatic system.

. . . .

. . . .

. . . .

19. Briefly describe the pathway of lymph from lymph capillaries to the subclavian veins (include lymph nodes).

. . . .

. . . .

. . . .

. . . .

. . . .

20. What parts do the central nervous system consist of?

. . . .

21. What is the peripheral nervous system? Give examples of nerves found within it.

. . . .

. . . .

. . . .

22. Briefly describe the autonomic nervous system.

. . . .

. . . .

. . . .

23. List **3** endocrine glands and state a hormone each releases and its function.

. . . .

. . . .

. . . .

24. Briefly describe gas exchange within the lungs.

. . . .

. . . .

. . . .

25. Why should gentle pressure be used when giving abdominal massage?

. . . .

. . . .

. . . .

26. Name **4** parts that make up the urinary system.

. . . .

. . . .

27. Why should gentle pressure be used when massaging over the kidney areas?

. . . .

. . . .

. . . .

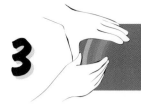

THE PROFESSIONAL THERAPIST

The therapist needs to present a professional image and manner when carrying out body massage treatment. If the first impression is bad it is unlikely the client will return for further treatment.

A therapist should:

- wear a clean and ironed overall, either a dress or a tunic top and trousers
- wear clean shoes with a low heel
- tie back long hair, which should be clean
- have short, clean nails
- wear little or no jewellery. If a watch or bracelet is worn it may scratch the client during the massage
- have a high standard of personal hygiene
- be friendly and approachable.

PREPARING THE TREATMENT ROOM

The therapy room should be clean, tidy and well presented. Ensure everything is at hand and towels are folded, the trolley neatly laid out, with perhaps crystals and an attractive bowl to pour out the oil. You may also consider subdued lighting and relaxing music. There needs to be adequate heating because if clients are cold they will not enjoy the massage.

Equipment and materials

The trolley and couch must be set up before the client comes for treatment.

Below is a checklist to help you prepare. Ensure you have the following.

1 Client consultation form and pen.

2 Large and small clean towels laid on to the couch and some on bottom tier of trolley.

3 Couch roll placed on to the trolley and couch.

4 Clean gown for the client.

5 Blanket, in case the client becomes cold.

6 Bolsters and/or rolled-up towels.

7 CD player to play relaxing music.

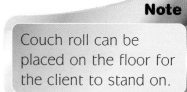

Note

Couch roll can be placed on the floor for the client to stand on.

The trolley should contain the following items:

♦ massage mediums. If using cream disposable spatulas should be used

♦ bowls for client's jewellery and cotton wool

♦ surgical spirit or antiseptic solution to clean the feet

♦ eau-de-cologne to wipe off excess oil if required

♦ tissues.

Using a pencil and the equipment and materials checklist on page 99, set up the treatment room below in preparation for the client's arrival.

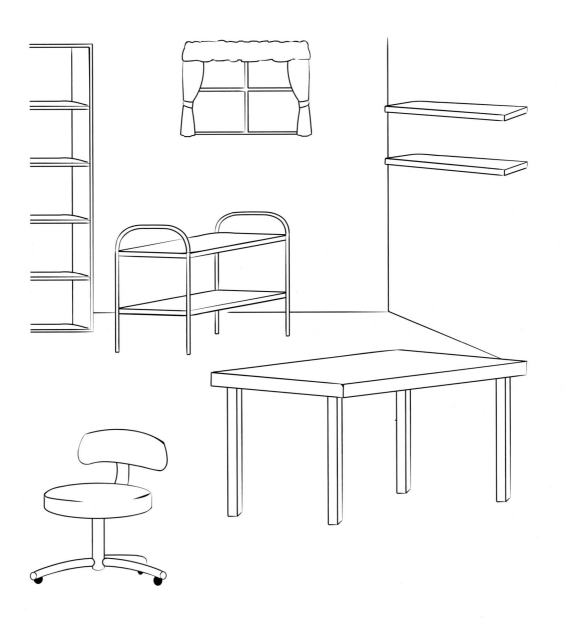

Figure 3.1   *The treatment room*

How long will the treatment take?

A body massage treatment will last for about one hour and the consultation will take 15 minutes. A back massage will take about 20 minutes.

Note

Ensure your client is aware of how long the treatment will take and how much it will cost.

CONSULTATION

The consultation is an important part of the massage treatment and lasts for about 15 minutes, although the first consultation may take longer. It begins with greeting the client and asking him or her to sit down. Ensure you smile often and give regular eye contact so the client feels at ease in your company. During the consultation ask open-ended questions, using words such as 'what' and 'how'. You will gain a lot more information from the client.

A consultation form is used to write down client information; inform the client that all information given is confidential and that the details will be securely stored. Ensuring client confidentiality will help create a trusting professional relationship between the client and therapist.

Note

Ensure any possessions are safely stored during treatment.

Be aware of your non-verbal communication and also look at the client's non-verbal communication, e.g. is there nervousness, but most importantly you should listen carefully to what the client has to say. The consultation is essential for the following reasons:

- you can develop a good relationship with the client
- to find out if there are any medical reasons (contra-indications) that would prevent the treatment being carried out
- what the client's expectations of the treatment are, which will also help to reassure a nervous client
- it helps you to treat the client in a holistic way as you can find out about the lifestyle of the client;

Note

The term holistic is derived from the Greek word 'Holos' meaning whole.

perhaps emotional factors are causing persistent aches and pains. Maybe their job involves bending the neck a great deal so causing neck problems or perhaps heavy lifting is affecting the shoulders. If the client feels persistently tired, often a cause of this is stress, and so breathing and relaxation techniques can be given

◆ you can discuss the treatment plan, duration and the cost of the treatment with the client.

Ensure that clients understand exactly what the massage entails and that you, as the therapist, understand their expectations.

Note

Make a note of points of interest discussed by clients, perhaps an exam, holiday, wedding, etc. You can ask how they got on the next time you meet.

Task 3.2

Think of 10 ways in which you could help ensure client satisfaction when giving massage treatment, e.g. be punctual.

Opposite is an example of a body massage consultation form. It is important that you discuss any contra-indications with the client, but if there are questions on the form that you feel are too personal to discuss on the first consultation, you can ask these questions on the next visit instead. Always ensure the client reads the client declaration and signs the consultation form!

BODY MASSAGE CONSULTATION FORM

NAME: **TEL NO:**
ADDRESS:

EMAIL ADDRESS:
D.O.B: **OCCUPATION:**

MEDICAL QUESTIONNAIRE
Do you suffer from or have suffered from any of the following?
High or low blood pressure? ....
Heart condition? ....
Liver complaints (e.g. hepatitis)? ....
Epilepsy? ....
Digestive problems (e.g. irritable bowel syndrome)? ....
Recent haemorrhage? ....
Thrombosis or embolism? ....
Lumps/swellings? ....
Varicose veins? ....
Diabetes? ....
Spastic conditions (e.g. muscular spasms)? ....
Dysfunction of the nervous system (e.g. Parkinson's disease)? ....
Skin disorders/scalp infections? ....
Allergies/sensitive skin? ....
Cuts or abrasions in area being treated? ....
Recent operations? ....
Fluid retention (oedema)? ....
Any discomfort/pain in your body? ....
Anxiety/depression? ....
Any other health problems or recent illnesses? ....
Current medication? ....

Are you pregnant? ....
Is GP referral required? Yes/No ....
Name of doctor: ....
Surgery address and tel no: ....

LIFESTYLE

Do you drink alcohol, if so how often? ....

Do you smoke, if so how many each day?...

Do you eat healthily? ....

Do you drink plenty of fluids (water)?..

Do you sleep well? ....

How often do you exercise? ....

What are your hobbies, how do you relax?..

Are you going through any major life changes such as menopause, bereavement, loss of job, retirement, etc? ....

Would you say your stress levels are: high/average/low?

Details if levels are high:

Would you say your energy levels are: high/average/poor?

Any previous holistic therapy treatments?

Why have you come for massage treatment?

Additional notes:

(e.g. Is there any referral data from other health professionals?)

Client declaration

The information I have given regarding my medical details is accurate. I will promptly notify the therapist of any future changes to my health.

Client signature ....Date ....

Treatment notes/homecare advice given

Figure 3.2   *Body massage consultation form*

When clients come for the next treatment you do not need to complete another form. However, you will need to find out if their circumstances have changed in any way since the last treatment, especially medically, and note it on their form. Any client records kept on computer must comply with the Data Protection Act (see Chapter 8).

CONTRA-INDICATIONS

Body massage is a very safe treatment. However, there are certain conditions that the therapist should be aware of, which may prevent treatment being carried out or require the advice of a doctor. The contra-indications to massage are:

- high blood pressure/low blood pressure
- thrombosis/embolism
- phlebitis
- recent operations
- any recent fractures or sprains
- severe bruising, cuts or abrasion in treatment area
- epilepsy
- recent haemorrhage or swellings
- diabetes
- spastic conditions
- dysfunction of the nervous system
- skin disorders/nail diseases/scalp infections
- varicose veins
- pregnancy

- first two days of menstruation on abdomen
- sunburn
- fever
- infectious diseases
- cancer.

Some of these conditions are known as local contra-indications, such as bruises and varicose veins. They can be worked around and do not necessarily mean that massage treatment cannot be carried out. General contra-indications such as diabetes and epilepsy may require advice from the client's doctor before treatment can be given. The contra-indications are discussed in more detail below.

If during consultation clients inform you, for instance, they have a thrombosis so are contra-indicated to treatment, it should be explained to clients that it is in their interests not to continue with treatment, as it could potentially harm them or worsen their condition.

High blood pressure (HBP)

High blood pressure (hypertension) is when the blood pressure is consistently higher than normal. It occurs when there is an increase in the force of blood flow against the artery and heart walls. Smoking, obesity, lack of exercise, eating too much salt, stress, too much alcohol, the contraceptive pill, pregnancy and heredity are all contributing factors. There are no obvious symptoms of high blood pressure, but it can lead to strokes and heart attacks as the heart has to work harder to force blood through the system.

Massage increases the blood circulation thus possibly increasing the blood pressure, but as vasodilation (widening) of the blood vessels also occurs massage could have the effect of lowering the blood pressure, especially after a while. These effects probably counterbalance each other. Massage treatment is also relaxing, so can also be of benefit to people with high blood pressure that has been brought on by stress. Abnormal blood pressure is an important contra-indication and it is advisable to seek the doctor's advice.

Note

Clients on anti-hypertensive drugs to help treat high blood pressure may suffer with postural hypotension (low blood pressure), so when they stand up after treatment they may feel light headed and dizzy.

Low blood pressure (LBP)

Low blood pressure (hypotension) is when the blood pressure is below normal for a substantial time. Blood pressure must be sufficient to pump blood to the brain when the body is in the upright position. If it is not then the person will feel faint. It is advisable to seek the advice of a doctor before treatment.

Advise clients suffering with HBP or LBP to get up slowly after treatment. For clients suffering with HBP ensure the treatment is relaxing by using lots of stroking movements. It is also recommended that the back of the couch is slightly raised during treatment.

History of thrombosis or embolism

A blood clot (thrombus) forms within an artery or vein, gradually blocking the flow of blood. The clot may be formed by sluggish blood flow or an accumulation of fats in the blood. It is dangerous as it may constrict or cut off the flow of blood. If massage is carried out there is a risk that the clot (thrombus) may be moved or broken up and taken to the heart, lungs or brain, which could prove fatal. Thrombosis that occurs in the deep veins is known as deep vein thrombosis (DVT), and often forms in the legs.

Embolism is a blockage of an artery with a clot of material that is contained within the bloodstream. The blockage can be due to a number of things, including a thrombus, air, fat or even bone marrow. It circulates the bloodstream until it becomes wedged somewhere in a blood vessel and blocks the flow of blood. Such a blockage may be extremely harmful. Do not treat clients with thrombosis or embolism, and if there has been a history of these conditions obtain the doctor's advice.

Phlebitis

Phlebitis is inflammation of the veins and often accompanies thrombosis. Clients should be referred to their doctor.

Recent operations

If the client has had any recent operations on an area that you intend to treat, especially within the last six months, it is wise not to carry out the massage treatment or if possible massage around the affected area. If the operation is minor, the doctor's advice can be sought.

Any recent fractures or sprains

Massage would be extremely uncomfortable for a client and could worsen the condition. The area must be fully healed before treatment can take place.

Severe bruising, cuts or abrasions in treatment area

Bruises, cuts and abrasions are localised contra-indications, so massage can be carried out around them. If bruising or cuts are severe it may be wise to ask the client to return after the affected area has healed. If there is slight bleeding ensure that a plaster covers the infected area and that you do not touch it in case of cross-infection.

Note

Do not touch anything contaminated with blood unless you have surgical gloves on. Put the item into a plastic bag and tie the top to secure it. Ensure the bag and gloves are disposed of safely.

Epilepsy

Epilepsy is a disorder of the brain in which the patient suffers fits or seizures. The seizures are due to an excessive electrical discharge from nerve cells in the brain. The seizures may be partial, and the sufferer is still conscious, or general, where consciousness is lost. Usually there is no obvious cause, however, in some cases the fits could be due to scars on the brain from surgery or injury. If the epilepsy is controlled by medication the chances of seizure during a massage treatment are minimal. The advice of a doctor should be sought before treatment can be carried out.

Recent haemorrhage or swellings

Haemorrhage is the term for excessive bleeding, which can be internal or external. It is advisable not to give treatment to someone who has had a recent haemorrhage because the massage may cause further haemorrhaging.

Diabetes

Diabetes mellitus results when the body produces very little or no insulin from a gland called the pancreas. Insulin is needed to allow glucose (sugar) into the body's cells so the body can use it to make energy. The lack of insulin causes the sugar to build up in the blood instead. Some symptoms indicating diabetes include tiredness, an initial weight loss and excessive thirst and urination.

People with poorly controlled diabetes may have related conditions such as high blood pressure, hardened arteries, altered sensations in limbs such as numbness, eyesight problems, poor healing of the skin and wasting of the tissues, such as the skin, which may be paper thin and easily broken. Massage would need to be gentle. It is advisable to seek the advice of the doctor before treatment.

Spastic conditions

When the muscles are in spasm, so in a state of contraction, massage could be uncomfortable to the client. Spasms of the skeletal muscles often occur as a result of tissue damage, perhaps due to injury or emotional stress. There is a build-up of toxins in the muscles, which irritate the nerves and lead to pain.

Dysfunction of the nervous system

Any dysfunction of the nervous system includes conditions such as multiple sclerosis, cerebral palsy, Parkinson's disease and motor neurone disease. The doctor's advice should be sought prior to treatment.

Skin disorders/nail diseases/scalp infections

Treatment can be given if the skin disorder, nail disease or scalp infection is not infectious, there is no bleeding or weeping and would not cause discomfort to the client when massaged. Otherwise the area can be worked around or the client should return when the condition has cleared.

Varicose veins

Varicose veins are blue, prominent and permanently dilated (widened) veins in which blood pools, causing them to swell and bulge. They are due to valves in the veins not working properly and commonly occur in the veins near the surface of the leg and also in the anus (haemorrhoids). The condition is often made worse by pregnancy, the menopause, obesity and long periods of standing. A thrombosis can sometimes occur within a varicose vein. A varicose vein is a local contra-indication so massage treatment can be given around the affected area.

Pregnancy

Pregnancy can lead to a variety of contra-indications such as high blood pressure so only those therapists who have a full understanding of the specific contra-indications that pregnancy can cause, and feel confident to do so, should perform any treatment on pregnant clients. Before any treatment can be carried out the client's doctor or midwife's advice should be sought.

Note

Ensure your insurance covers you to work on pregnant women.

First two days of menstruation on the abdomen

The abdomen will be tender at this time so no massage should be given on the abdomen, although the rest of the body may be massaged.

Cancer

It is feared that giving massage treatment to someone suffering with cancer will cause the cancer to spread through the lymphatic and circulatory systems, although there has been no evidence to support this. Massage may be given if under medical supervision.

Note

Check with your insurance company to ensure you are covered to give massage to people with cancer.

Note

Ask clients to obtain their doctor's advice if you are ever unsure whether it is safe to give a treatment!

Task 3.3

How many contra-indications to massage can you remember? List them below:

REFERRAL LETTER TO CLIENT'S DOCTOR

If clients have a contra-indication it is advisable they obtain advice from their doctor regarding their medical condition and suitability for treatment. A standard letter can be given to their doctor or posted enclosing a stamped addressed envelope. The doctor need only sign their name to advise their patient if they think there is a medical reason why treatment should not go ahead.

Note

Ensure you also send a leaflet, which briefly explains the treatment, as the doctor may not know what a body massage treatment entails!

Address of treatment room

Date ....

Dear Dr [name]

Your patient, [name] of [his/her address] has informed me that he/she is suffering from [high blood pressure, diabetes, etc].

Please advise me if in your view there is any reason why your patient should not have body massage treatment.

Thank you

Yours sincerely

[Your signature]
[Your name printed]

Doctor's advice

I feel [name of client] would/would not be suitable for having massage treatment.

Doctor's signature .... Date........................

Figure 3.3 *Sample letter to doctor*

Doctors do not often know what a massage treatment entails and therefore cannot give permission as such for treatment to go ahead, only advise their patient. A doctor's insurance does not cover them for giving permission or consent regarding holistic therapy treatments.

HANDLING REFERRAL DATA FROM PROFESSIONAL SOURCES

If a health care professional, be it a doctor or a reflexologist, etc, should refer a client to you for massage treatment, it is courteous to keep them informed of the client's progress. A progress report should include the following information:

- the client's name, who referred them and their reason for coming for massage treatment
- the client's progress
- treatment plan for the future.

A brief letter can be written reporting the progress of a client, an example of which follows.

Note

Ensure you have the client's permission before sending the progress report.

Date

Salon address

Dear Dr Douglas
Thank you for recommending Sara Beattie of 25 Orville Terrace, Bruton to come for massage treatment. I am writing to inform you of her progress.

Sara has been having regular weekly treatments for the past month to help treat her back problem. She feels that the treatments have helped ease the muscle stiffness in her back and as a result is experiencing less discomfort.

We are to continue her treatments for two more weeks and she will return to me on a monthly basis.

If you require further information please do not hesitate to contact me.

Yours sincerely

Ms F. Gould

Figure 3.4 *Sample progress letter to doctor*

PREPARING A TREATMENT PLAN

A treatment plan will ensure you have a plan of action, which will help you and your client reach your objectives. The plan will include the client's expectations of the treatment, therefore helping to ensure client satisfaction.

At any time you can change your treatment plan to suit you and your client. You can also monitor progress to see if changes are needed in any way.

How often should a client come for treatment?

You will need to discuss how often the treatment should be carried out with your clients. It will depend on their finances, time and their reasons for coming. If they have come for relaxation maybe they could attend once every two weeks; if they have a particular condition that needs treating you could advise coming for treatment once a week for five weeks. Emphasise to your client the importance of regular treatments to maintain the long-term benefits.

Below is an example of a treatment plan.

Client name Ms F. Willets   **Date of treatment** Dec 30th

Treatment given   Holistic body massage

What are the client's expectations of treatment?
- To ease discomfort and pain she is suffering in her back
- To be relaxed.

What are the treatment objectives?
- To release muscular tension in the lower back to decrease pain and discomfort experienced by client. Use lots of effleurage and petrissage movements to encourage blood and lymph circulation to muscles of back and buttocks.
- To relax the client, so use mainly effleurage movements and avoid tapotement.

Medium chosen and amount used sweet almond (20 ml)

Recommended frequency of treatment
Weekly treatments for a period of five weeks (this can be changed at a later date).

Additional notes:
- Any preference to medium used
- Any areas client does not want massaged
- Particular areas of tension in body that need specific massage
- Any fluid retention
- Postural assessment
- Particular massage movements enjoyed by client
- Any special needs, maybe need help on to couch, use of pillows/bolsters
- Outcome of treatment, was it effective?
- Any problems that arise.

Figure 3.5 *Treatment plan*

Note

Write to your client's husband or wife a couple of weeks before your client's birthday and ask if he or she would like to buy a voucher for a massage treatment.

EVALUATION OF TREATMENT

It is important to evaluate the massage treatment given to the client. How could you have improved the treatment? Ask the client questions such as 'Did you enjoy the treatment?'. A client feedback form may be given to a client to fill in; it will help establish which aspects of the treatment may need improvement. An example is given below.

Client feedback form

It is our aim to provide a professional service and we value your opinion regarding the massage treatment. It would be appreciated if you would answer the following questions. You do not have to write your name if you prefer.

Client name: Date:

Was the therapist friendly and professional?   Yes   No

If no, please comment

. . . .

Was the treatment room clean, warm and inviting?   Yes   No

If no, please comment

Did the treatment meet with your expectations?   Yes   No

If no, please comment

Would you book another massage treatment?   Yes   No

If no, please comment

Are there any additional comments you would like to make regarding the treatment?

Client signature ....   Date ....

Figure 3.6   *Client feedback form*

1. Why is it important for the therapist to be well presented and to have a professional attitude?

   . . . .

   . . . .

   . . . .

2. Why must particular attention be paid to personal and general hygiene when treating clients?

   . . . .

   . . . .

   . . . .

3. Why is it important to be aware of the client's body language (perhaps they are nervous) and how would you reassure them about the massage treatment?

   . . . .

   . . . .

   . . . .

4. How could you make a client feel at ease and relaxed in your company during the consultation?

   . . . .

   . . . .

   . . . .

5. State three reasons why giving a consultation is so important.

   . . . .

   . . . .

   . . . .

6. Name **five** things you could do to ensure the safety of yourself, your client and possessions during treatment.

. . . .

. . . .

. . . .

. . . .

. . . .

7. List **six** contra-indications to massage treatment.

. . . .

. . . .

. . . .

. . . .

. . . .

. . . .

8. If during the consultation your client informs you that he or she has a general contra-indication what action would you take?

. . . .

. . . .

. . . .

9. Why is it important to establish the reasons the client has come to you and their expectations during the consultation?

. . . .

. . . .

. . . .

10. Why should the client record card be clearly written and all the information be accurate and regularly updated?

....

....

....

11. What is the purpose of a treatment plan?

....

....

....

12. Why is it important to evaluate the massage treatment?

....

....

....

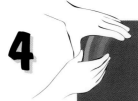

Massage Techniques and Preparing for Massage Treatment

4

ASSESSING THE CLIENT'S POSTURE

Assessing the client's posture prior to body massage treatment will help you identify any postural faults. Massage can be helpful for postural problems and corrective exercises may be given as part of the aftercare advice.

A good posture means that the body is aligned and balanced, so that muscles only need to carry out minimum work to maintain it. It will ensure muscles and joints are working efficiently so that the body remains free from muscular tension, strains, stiffness and pain. Good posture will help encourage efficient breathing and aid digestion, as the organs will not be compressed or restricted due to bad posture and tightened muscles.

Posture is influenced by various factors including the following:

- tension and stress
- illness
- hereditary factors
- adopting a poor posture when standing or sitting
- pregnancy
- height and weight of individual
- age of individual.

To evaluate a posture a plumb line may be used to check the alignment of the body; a weight tied on to the end of a piece of string can be used. Clients should wear their underwear and stand with shoulders relaxed and arms by their sides. First, observe the client from the front.

- Are the ear lobes level? If not, the sternocleidomastoid and upper area of the trapezius muscle could be tight on the side that the ear lobe is highest and the muscles on the other side stretched.

- Is one shoulder higher than the other? If so, the upper area of the trapezius and levator scapulae muscles are tight on the shoulder that is higher.

- Are both shoulders lifted and held high? Stress and tension often cause tightening of the trapezius and levator scapulae muscles.

- Are the waist and hips level each side? If not, there may be a spinal defect or one leg may be shorter than the other.

- Is one leg shorter than the other? This may indicate scoliosis or another spinal condition so there may be associated muscular pain and stiffness.

- Do the feet point outwards? This may indicate flat feet, where there is flattening of the medial arch.

Observe the client from the side. The plumb line should pass the lobe of the ear, the shoulder joint, the hip joint, behind the patella and just in front of the protruding ankle bone.

- Does the chin poke forward? This may indicate a postural fault called kyphosis.

- Is the abdomen protruding and pelvis tilting forward? This may mean the abdominal muscles are overstretched and weak. It could indicate there is a postural fault called lordosis.

Note

Occasionally a client may show signs of kyphosis *and* lordosis.

Observe the client from the back.

◆ Is the spine straight? If there is a 's' or 'c' shape curve to the spine it may indicate a postural fault called scoliosis.

◆ Are the buttocks sagging? This will indicate that the gluteal muscles are weak.

CORRECTION OF POSTURE

To help correct a posture take into account the following points:

◆ the client's head should be up with chin in

◆ shoulders back, but down and relaxed

◆ abdominal muscles pulled in

◆ buttock muscles tightened and tucked in

◆ knees slightly bent

◆ weight of body evenly distributed on both feet.

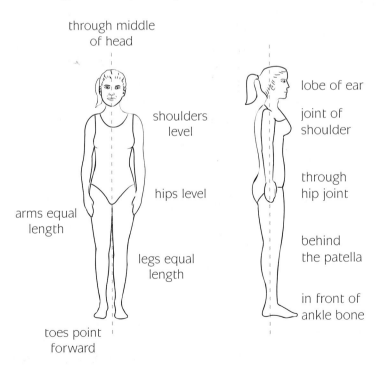

Figure 4.1 *Assessing and correcting the posture*

POSTURAL FAULTS

A poor posture means that the body is out of balance so that certain muscles have to contract strongly to maintain it. Over a period of time these muscles will tighten and shorten, while other muscles will stretch and weaken. Three main postural faults are lordosis, kyphosis and scoliosis.

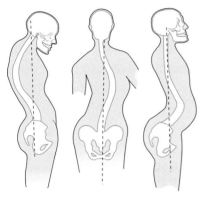

Kyphosis   Scoliosis   Lordosis

Figure 4.2   *Posture faults*

Lordosis

Lordosis is a condition that shows itself as an inward exaggeration of the lumbar region of the spine. The client will appear to have a hollow back and there will be protrusion of the abdomen and buttocks. Gymnasts often adopt this posture.

- Weak muscles: the hamstrings, gluteus maximus, rectus abdominis, internal and external oblique muscles are stretched and lengthened.

- Tight muscles: the muscles of the lumbar region are shortened.

Corrective exercises for lordosis

Ensure the client is safely able to undertake exercise and that there are no contra-indications.

1 The client should lie on their back with legs bent, feet flat on the floor and arms by his or her side. The lumbar region of the spine is pushed into the floor and then released. This exercise is repeated six times and will help to stretch the lower back muscles.

2 In the same position, with the chin tucked in, the head and shoulders are lifted to look at the knees. Repeat this exercise six times. This exercise will help to strengthen the abdominal muscles.

3 In the same position but with the hands resting behind the head, alternately bring the elbows to touch the opposite knee. Repeat six times to each side. This exercise will help to strengthen the oblique muscles.

Kyphosis

Kyphosis is a condition where there is an exaggeration of the thoracic curve of the spine. The client will have rounded shoulders and the chin often pokes forwards.

- Weak muscles: the upper back muscles are weakened and overstretched.
- Tight muscles: the pectoral muscles are tightened and shortened.
- Adopting a poor posture often causes kyphosis.

Corrective exercises for kyphosis

The client should stand for all the following exercises; ensure that he or she has a good posture. Each exercise should be repeated six times.

1 Pull the shoulders backwards, hold for three seconds and then release.

2 Circle the shoulders backwards, hold for three seconds and then release.

3 Alternately circle the arms backwards.

These exercises will help to strengthen the upper back muscles and stretch out the muscles of the chest.

Note

Effleurage and petrissage techniques will also help to stretch the muscles that are tight.

Scoliosis

A sign of scoliosis is a curvature of the spine, which may be C or S shaped. It can result in the level of the shoulders and pelvic girdle being slightly uneven. An individual may be born with this condition or other factors such as the continual carrying of heavy bags on one particular shoulder over a period of time can cause it. The muscles which are shortened and tight are found on the inside of the curve, and the muscles which are overstretched will be found on the outside of the curve. Shortened and tight muscles can be relaxed and stretched with massage so can help to correct posture faults.

Corrective exercises for scoliosis

1 The client should be stride standing. Using the hand on the side of the curve where the muscles are shortened, reach it straight into the air. The other arm should be stretched so that the hand reaches towards the floor. Release the stretch and repeat six times. This exercise will help to stretch the shortened and tight muscles.

2 The client should be stride standing, with arms at each side. Ask him or her to flex the side of the trunk where the muscles are overstretched. Repeat six times. This exercise will help to strengthen the muscles that are overstretched.

Complete the table by naming the overstretched and tight muscles associated with each postural fault and briefly describe one corrective exercise for each.

Table 4.1 Postural faults and corrective exercises

Postural fault	Overstretched muscles	Tight muscles	Briefly describe one corrective exercise
Lordosis			
Kyphosis			
Scoliosis			

WORKING POSTURES

There are two types of working postures used throughout the massage. These postures will help prevent strain and injury.

Figure 4.3
Working postures

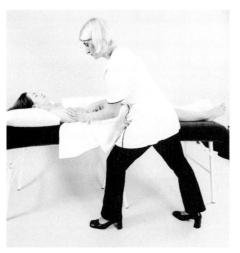

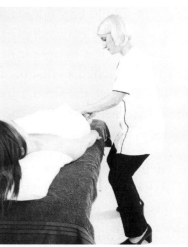

♦ Walk standing: stand with feet apart, place one foot in front of the other as if walking. This stance is used when massaging up and down the length of the body.

♦ Stride standing: stand with both feet apart, facing forwards. This stance is used when working across the body.

MASSAGE TECHNIQUES

The four main types of massage techniques are:

- effleurage
- petrissage
- tapotement, also known as percussion
- vibrations.

Each massage technique consists of various massage movements.

Table 4.2 The various massage movements

Effleurage	Petrissage	Tapotement	Vibrations
Stroking	Kneading	Hacking	Shaking
Effleurage	Frictions	Cupping	Vibrations
	Picking up	Beating	
	Wringing	Pounding	
	Knuckling		
	Skin rolling		

Effleurage

Stroking

Stroking is a gentle and slow movement (as when stroking a cat or dog) and involves the smooth gliding of the hands over a body part. It is mostly a restful movement, ideal to use at the beginning or the end of the massage. One hand or both hands can be used and either the palm of the hand or tips of the fingers or thumbs can be used to perform this movement. Stroking is often carried out on the back and can be performed in any direction.

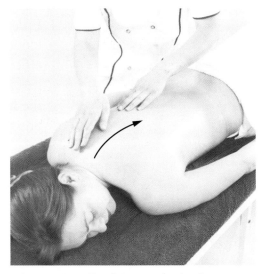

Figure 4.4 *Stroking to the back*

Effects of stroking on the body

♦ Induces relaxation.

♦ Calming to the nerves.

♦ Lightly stimulates blood circulation.

♦ Lightly stimulates lymphatic circulation.

Uses of stroking

♦ To calm and relax.

♦ To create erythema and warm up an area.

♦ To use over the abdomen to help prevent or treat constipation.

Effleurage

Effleurage is similar to, although a deeper movement than, stroking and is usually performed slowly. Effleurage can be superficially or deeply applied to the body. The hands may be used alternately or both together to perform this massage movement. The hands must completely relax and mould to the shape of the limb or part treated.

Note

Effleurage is a French word meaning 'stroking'.

Effleurage should be carried out in the same direction as blood travels in the veins, known as venous return, e.g. effleurage should be applied in an upward direction on the legs and arms, in the direction of the heart. At the end of the movement the hands glide back using almost no pressure at all.

On areas such as the face, fingers and toes, the pads of the fingertips or thumb may be used to effleurage the area instead of the whole hand.

How to perform effleurage

1 Adopt the walk standing position.

2 Ensure fingers and thumbs of each hand are placed together, in contact with each other.

3 With the back straight and the front knee bent, place your hands on to the area to be massaged.

4 Begin to massage using the whole palmar surface of the hands, ensuring the hands are relaxed and mould to the body part as they slide along.

5 Make sure that the hands maintain contact on the return stroke, although the pressure will be light.

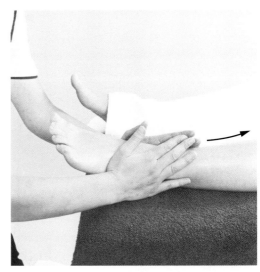

Figure 4.5   *Effleurage to the leg*

Effects of effleurage on the body

◆ Promotes relaxation.

◆ Has a soothing effect on the nerves.

◆ Increases blood flow.

◆ Increases lymphatic flow.

◆ Stimulates sebaceous glands so more sebum is produced.

◆ Stimulates sweat glands so more sweat is produced.

Uses of effleurage

◆ To begin and end massage on a body part.

◆ To warm the skin and prepare the muscles for deeper work (similar to a warm-up prior to undertaking exercise).

- To link one massage movement with another to help the massage flow smoothly.

- To help spread the oil or cream over the area to be massaged.

- To promote relaxation.

- To improve lymphatic drainage, so is useful for fluid retention.

- To improve venous (blood in veins) drainage.

- To help eliminate toxins from an area after stimulating movements such as tapotement have been used.

Petrissage

Note

Petrissage is a French word meaning 'kneading'.

Petrissage movements involve deeper pressure than those used for effleurage and are useful for working deep into the muscle tissue. These movements usually involve pressing the muscle against the bone or lifting it away from the bone. Massage movements for the petrissage group include kneading, frictions, picking up, wringing, skin rolling and knuckling.

Kneading

There are different types of kneading massage movements, including palmar kneading, thumb kneading and finger kneading.

- Palmar kneading: the palm of one hand (single handed) or both (double handed) is used to create fairly deep circular movements. The pressure is mainly applied during the upward part of the circle. There are different types of palmar kneading, which include single handed kneading, double handed kneading, alternate palmar kneading and reinforced palmar kneading.

- Single handed kneading: as the name suggests, only one hand is used to massage, the other can rest elsewhere on the body.

- Double handed kneading: both hands are used to knead an area.

- Reinforced palmar kneading: one hand is placed on top of the other to produce a deeper pressure.

How to perform kneading

1 Mould your hand to the shape of the body part to be massaged.

2 If you are using the right hand, create circles in a clockwise direction. The circles can be applied in an anti-clockwise direction if using the left hand.

3 From the bottom to the top of each circle apply pressure and from the top to the bottom of each circle you can release pressure to complete the circle.

4 You can work in any direction on the body but remember to work up the limbs towards the direction of the heart.

- Thumb kneading: the pads of the thumbs are used to perform fairly deep and small circular movements. These movements can be used on most parts of the body except bony areas or areas with little muscle tissue. Thumb kneading is useful for treating muscular tension and to break down knots within muscle.

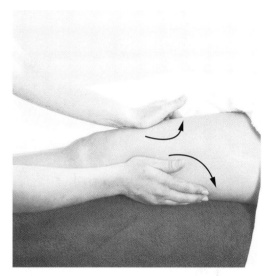

Figure 4.6a   *Double handed palmar kneading*

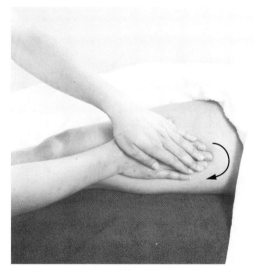

Figure 4.6b   *Reinforced palmar kneading*

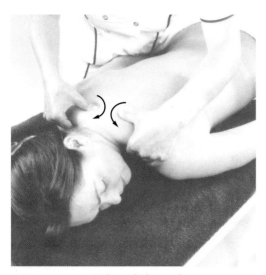

Figure 4.7   *Thumb kneading*

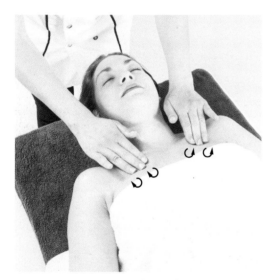

Figure 4.8   *Finger kneading*

◆ Finger kneading: with the fingers close together use the pads to create fairly deep and small circular movements. Finger kneading is particularly useful around the joints of the ankles, over the pectorals, either side of the spine and around the colon.

Frictions

Friction comes from a Latin word, *fricare*, which means to rub. Hence, friction techniques are all forms of rubbing. They are performed with the fingers or thumb and used on specific localised areas. They are deep movements performed with much pressure and are useful for breaking down 'knots' and loosening tightness in muscles. When performed on either side of the spine it will stimulate spinal nerves and help to invigorate the client. Frictions should be performed on dry skin, so any oil or cream should be removed.

How to perform frictions

1   Begin by stroking the area with the palm or thumb and then place the middle finger on the index finger.

2   Create tiny circles with these fingers, applying deeper and deeper pressure into the tissues and then release. This movement can be repeated three times and then another area can be worked.

3   Stroke over the area with the fingers or thumb to soothe.

Note

Fast stroking or rubbing with the whole hand is sometimes known as friction. It is a different movement to 'frictions' as the pressure is fairly light and a larger area can be worked over.

Picking up

The tissues are picked up, lifted way from the bone, squeezed and then released. One or both hands can be used. There are three main types: single handed picking up, double handed picking up and reinforced picking up.

● Single handed picking up: only one hand is used for this movement. It is ideal to use on areas such as the upper and lower arms.

How to perform single handed picking up

1 Make a C shape with your fingers and thumb.

2 Place your hand on to the area to be massaged.

3 Using the thumb and fingers, squeeze and lift away the muscle using a circular motion.

4 Release the muscle and slide the hand forwards. Repeat this movement until the whole muscle or body part has been worked.

● Double handed picking up: although similar to single handed picking up, both hands are used for this movement. It is ideal to use on large areas such as the back or thigh.

How to perform double handed picking up

1 With the elbows abducted, place both hands side by side on the body part, about 5 centimetres apart. Abduct the thumb away from the fingers. Using one hand only, pick up the tissues by sliding the fingers and thumbs towards each other so that the tissues are picked up and squeezed.

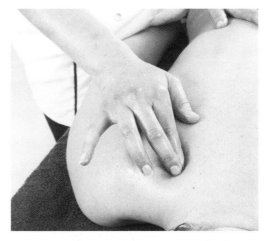

Figure 4.9   *Frictions to upper back*

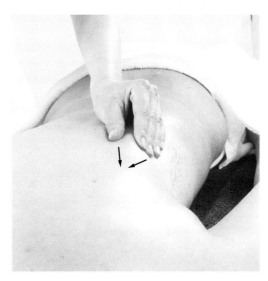

Figure 4.10   *Single handed picking up to back*

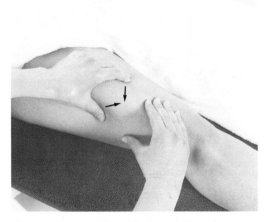

Figure 4.11 *Double handed picking up to leg*

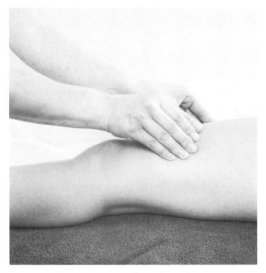

Figure 4.12 *Reinforced picking up to thigh*

2 As one hand releases the tissues, the other hand now lifts, squeezes and releases the tissues. The hands work alternately so a large area can be worked over.

◆ Reinforced picking up: this movement is similar to picking up but involves placing one hand on top of the other to increase the pressure and depth of the movement. It is often used on the thighs and back of the lower legs.

How to perform reinforced picking up

1 Abduct the thumbs and place one hand on top of the other so that each thumb is in contact with the index finger of the opposite hand. The right thumb will be hidden under the left index finger and the left thumb is on top of the right index finger. A 'V' shape is produced by the position of both hands.

2 The hands work together to pick up, squeeze and release the tissues.

Wringing

Wringing is a movement where the muscles are lifted away from the bone, and wrung from side to side as the hands move up and down across the length of the muscle. Both hands are used for this technique.

How to perform wringing

1 First, position the right hand forward of the other (see Figure 4.13). With both hands grasp the tissues between the fingers and thumbs.

2 With the tissues lifted and squeezed slide back the fingers of the right hand and push forward

the thumb of the left hand so that the right hand is sliding towards you and the left hand is sliding forwards. An 'S' shape is created with the tissues.

3 When you can no longer slide the hands, release the tissues. Now lift the tissues but this time pull the fingers of the left hand backwards and push forward the thumb of the right hand so that the right hand is sliding forwards and the left hand is sliding towards you.

This movement can be repeated many times working across the length of the muscle. It cannot be performed on areas with little tissue such as the ribs.

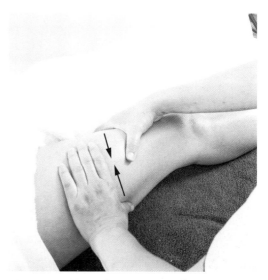

Figure 4.13a *Wringing to leg, one hand in front of other, squeezing*

Knuckling

This movement is excellent for working deep into the muscles and helps to relieve muscular tension. Do not use this movement over bony areas.

How to perform knuckling

1 Make a loose fist with your hand, the fingers and knuckles slightly apart.

2 Create circular movements with the fingers, using the parts of the fingers about 2.5 centimetres down from the nail to massage the area, and ensure the wrists are kept loose.

Skin rolling

This movement presses and rolls the skin and fat against the bone underneath. It is difficult to perform if there is little tissue present. It is often used on the back, sides of the trunk or across the limbs.

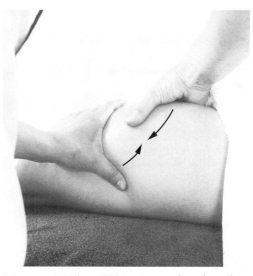

Figure 4.13b *Wringing to leg, hands coming back the other way*

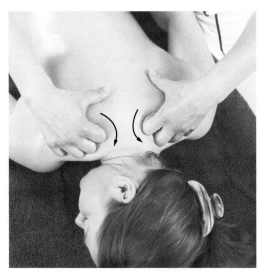

Figure 4.14 *Knuckling to back*

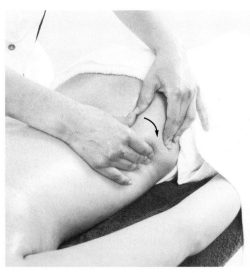

Figure 4.15 *Skin rolling to waist*

How to perform skin rolling

1 Create C shapes with both hands and press the fingers on to the skin, use the thumbs to push and roll the flesh towards the fingers.

2 Release and move the hands so that another area can be worked and repeat this movement.

Effects of petrissage on the body

◆ Increases blood circulation. Therefore brings fresh blood containing oxygen and nutrients to the area and removes waste products such as lactic acid that may be the cause of stiffness and discomfort in a muscle.

◆ Increases venous return (blood in the veins).

◆ Increases lymphatic flow so waste products and tissue fluid are removed more quickly. This will help with fluid retention (oedema).

◆ Stimulates blood supply to the bones and periosteum so fresh oxygen and nutrients will be delivered improving the health of the bone.

◆ Increased blood supply to the skin causes the cells in the basal layer to regenerate. As the cells divide they push upwards towards the surface of the skin. The dead skin cells of the horny layer will shed (desquamation), giving the skin a better texture and healthier look.

◆ Sweat glands are stimulated so more sweat is released helping to expel toxins.

◆ Sebaceous glands are stimulated to produce more sebum. This natural moisturiser will help keep the skin soft and moisturised.

◆ Stretches the muscles so improving their suppleness and elasticity.

◆ Helps to break down tension nodules (knots) within muscles.

Uses of petrissage

- To help relieve stiffness and pain in muscles as waste products will be removed from affected muscle.

- To help relieve constipation when massage is given to the abdomen in the direction of the colon.

- To stimulate poor blood circulation.

- To stimulate lymphatic drainage, therefore relieving fluid retention (oedema).

- To warm up muscles prior to exercise so that the muscles contract more easily. This will help to prevent injury and cramp occurring.

- To use before sport to warm the muscles so that flexibility is improved.

- To relax tense muscles and break down knots.

- To improve the condition of the skin so that it appears healthier looking.

Tapotement

Tapotement movements are also known as percussion movements. All tapotement movements are stimulating and so are usually left out of a relaxing massage. These movements should not be performed on bony areas, nor on old or very thin clients. Tapotement movements include hacking, cupping, beating and pounding, and are carried out at a fast pace.

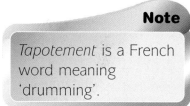

Note

Tapotement is a French word meaning 'drumming'.

Effects of tapotement on the body

- Increases blood circulation so produces erythema.

- Increases lymphatic flow.

- May help to increase muscle tone.

- Will help to stimulate and invigorate a client.

Uses of tapotement

- To improve sluggish blood circulation.

- To improve sluggish lymphatic circulation.
- To stimulate lethargic client.
- To improve muscle tone.
- To help improve cellulite conditions.

Hacking

This movement involves using the little finger, ring finger and the side of the hand, known as the ulnar border (because of the bone in the forearm called the ulna). The area worked is rapidly struck using alternate hands.

How to perform hacking

1 Place the little-finger sides of both hands, about 5 centimetres apart, on the area of the body to be massaged.

2 Fingers should not be completely straight but slightly cupped in shape.

3 With loose wrists, alternately chop with each hand, ensuring pressure is not too great.

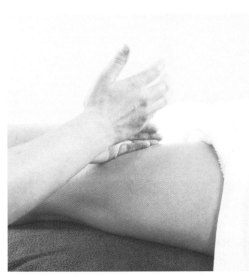

Figure 4.16 *Hacking to leg*

Note

Practise this movement on a pillow or cushion, as it can be quite difficult to master.

Cupping

Cupping is also known as clapping. As the name suggests the hands are cupped when performing this movement. The hands strike the body alternately, creating a hollow sound.

1 Cup both hands so that the fingers and thumb are close together and there are no gaps between them.

2 Alternately strike the body with both hands producing hollow sounds. Only the pads of the fingers and the bottom part of the palm will be in contact with the body.

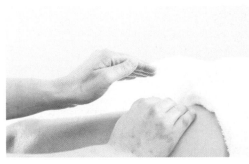

Figure 4.17 *Cupping to thigh*

Beating

This movement applies heavier pressure than the other tapotement techniques so it is good to use on areas of the body consisting of lots of adipose tissue (fat), such as the thighs and buttocks.

Note

Be careful not to slap the area, as this would be uncomfortable for the client.

How to perform beating

1 Loosely clench the fists with the thumbs tucked in, knuckles facing upwards.

2 With loose wrists alternately strike the area, applying deep pressure.

3 Work across the area until erythema (redness) is produced.

Pounding

Pounding also involves striking the body with loosely clenched fists but the ulnar border and little finger sides of both hands are used.

How to perform pounding

1 Loosely clench both fists with the thumb nails facing upwards.

2 The area will be pounded using the ulnar border (little finger) side of the hands.

3 Strike the body with one fist; as this fist lifts off the other fist will pound the area. The fists can circle each other, alternately pounding the skin.

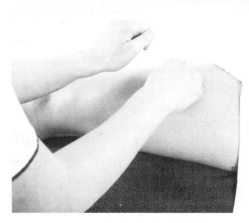

4 Work across the area until erythema is produced.

Figure 4.18 *Beating to thigh*

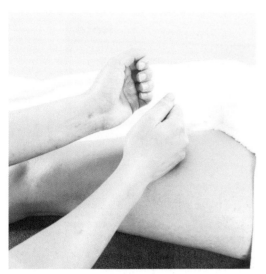

Figure 4.19 *Pounding to thigh*

Vibrations

The aim of vibration movements is to make the muscle shake so that tension can be released. There are two types of vibrations, namely shaking/rocking and vibrations.

Effects of vibration movements on the body

◆ Vibration movements are soothing to superficial nerves so relieve tension and induce relaxation.

◆ Vibration movements are useful to aid digestion and relieve flatulence when performed along the colon.

◆ Shaking movements help to relax the muscles, so relieve pain and stiffness.

Uses of vibrations

◆ Vibrations and shaking are used to relieve tension, relieve muscular pain and induce relaxation.

◆ Vibrations are used to help digestion and relieve flatulence.

◆ Shaking is used to relieve tension and stiffness in muscles.

◆ Vibrations and shaking will help to loosen fascia. Fascia is a sheath that covers muscles and extends to become tendons. Sometimes fascias of muscles stick together, therefore muscles cannot function as smoothly and these massage movements can be of great benefit.

Note

A similar movement to shaking is rocking. The whole hands can be used to gently rock a body part, such as a leg or the back.

Shaking

Shaking can be carried out on an arm or leg by grasping firmly around the ankle or wrist, lifting the limb and giving a gentle pull. The limb can be vigorously shaken, which will be stimulating for the client. If gently shaken it will be relaxing and sedating for the client.

Individual muscles or groups of muscles can be shaken, such as in the leg. The muscles are grasped and lifted between the thumb and fingers and gently shaken from side to side.

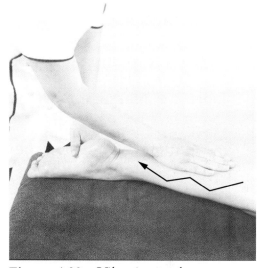

Figure 4.20 *Vibrations to leg*

Vibrations

This movement can be performed with one hand or both. The fingers, knuckles or whole of the hands can be used.

How to perform vibrations

1 Place one hand on to body and use the other hand to support the area.

2 The fingers should be straight, placed together with the thumb tucked in.

3 The hand can be vibrated side to side, which will create a shaking movement in the muscle.

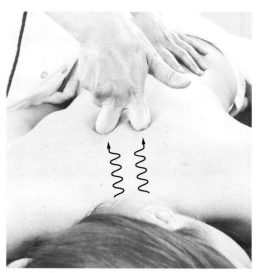

Figure 4.21 *Vibrations to either side of spine*

4 The working hand can remain in one position or move around so that different areas are worked.

5 On small areas such as down either side of the spine, the fingertips or knuckles can be used to vibrate.

Use the information given previously to complete Table 4.3.

Table 4.3 Massage movements

Massage movement	State if an effleurage, petrissage, tapotement or vibrations movement	Briefly describe a use and an effect of each massage movement
Cupping		
Effleurage		
Vibrations		
Frictions		
Picking up		
Pounding		
Knuckling		
Skin rolling		
Hacking		
Stroking		
Beating		
Wringing		
Shaking		
Rocking		
Kneading		

MEDIUMS

Most therapists choose to use a medium to carry out body massage treatment. Mediums commonly used include oil, creams and talc or arrowroot. All mediums should be applied to the therapist's hand and not directly on to the body. If the oil or cream is cold, gently rub between your hands to warm it up before applying on to the client.

Patch test

Although an allergic reaction to the oils is unusual, if a client has particularly sensitive skin a patch test can be carried out.

- Apply one drop of oil either behind the ear, on the inside of the wrist or at the crook of the arm. These are sensitive areas, which will respond well if there is going to be a reaction to the oil.

- The client should leave the area uncovered and unwashed for at least 24 hours.

- If the reaction is positive there will be redness, inflammation and itching and the client will probably find that he or she is scratching the area. If there is no reaction it is safe to use the oil.

Note

It is important to keep a record of the date and oils tested and state if there was a positive or negative reaction. Ensure that the client signs the record card.

Oil

It is recommended to use oils derived from plants such as grapeseed or olive oil. Although mineral oil is cheap, it has poor penetrative qualities so is not easily absorbed. It can clog the pores causing blackheads.

Oils are softening and nourishing to the skin and are particularly useful for dry skin. It is recommended to use about 25 millilitres of oil for a full body massage and 10 millilitres for a back massage. Additional oil may be needed if the client is large, has particularly dry skin or is generally hairy.

The oils should be unrefined, as the refining process means that the oils are extracted at high temperature resulting in nutrients being destroyed. This type of oil is often found on the supermarket shelves. The oils should be cold pressed and preferably free of additives, so look at the product label. Cold pressing involves pressing the nuts, kernels or seeds, etc with a hydraulic press so that the oil is squeezed out. Therefore oils retain their natural properties.

There are many oils that can be used for massage treatment and these include sweet almond, avocado, coconut, evening primrose, grapeseed, jojoba, olive, sunflower and wheatgerm.

Note

The oil molecules are too large to pass through the skin layers so mostly absorb into the upper layers of the skin and do not pass into the bloodstream.

Almond (sweet) oil

Sweet almond oil is extracted from the kernels of nuts belonging to the sweet almond tree. It is a pale yellow, thick liquid that mixes well with most other oils and essential oils. This popular oil is rich in nutrients such as unsaturated fatty acids, protein and vitamins A, B, D and E.

Uses of sweet almond

◆ Helps muscular tension, pain and stiffness.

◆ Excellent moisturiser for the skin.

◆ Helps to soothe and reduce inflammation.

◆ Beneficial for relieving itchiness associated with skin conditions such as eczema and psoriasis.

- Sweet almond is a safe oil to use but it is advisable not to use it on someone suffering from a nut allergy.

Avocado oil

The avocado tree is grown in many countries especially Spain. The oil is from the flesh of the avocado fruit and is green. It is solid at 0 degrees centigrade but liquefies at room temperature. The oil contains vitamins A, B1, B2 and D and many minerals including potassium, phosphorus, magnesium and calcium. It also contains proteins and fats. This oil is quite expensive so is often added to other oils.

Uses of avocado oil

- Excellent moisturiser for the skin.
- Penetrates deeper into the epidermis than most other oils.
- Has skin healing properties and helps reduce inflammation, so useful for conditions such as psoriasis and eczema.
- Helps to prevent premature ageing of the skin.

Coconut oil

The coconut palm tree is cultivated in many tropical areas such as Africa and South-East Asia. Coconut oil is a cream-coloured oil extracted from the dried flesh of the coconut. At room temperature coconut oil will be solid but will liquefy when warm. Placing the pot by a radiator or in warm water for a few minutes will warm and liquefy the oil.

Uses of coconut oil

- Softening and moisturising to the skin.
- Relieves inflamed skin.

Coconut oil can be used on its own or mixed with other oils. It may irritate sensitive skin so an allergy patch test should be given. It is advisable not to use it on someone with a nut allergy.

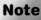

Note

Coconut oil is highly refined oil so many of the nutrients are destroyed during the refining process.

Evening primrose oil

The evening primrose plant is native to North America but is now common in the Mediterranean and is also grown in the UK. It is a plant with yellow-coloured flowers. Evening primrose oil is extracted from the seeds of the plant.

Uses of evening primrose oil

- Useful for dry, scaly skin.
- Helps wounds to heal.
- Useful for eczema.

It would be expensive to use this oil only. Evening primrose oil can be added to an oil in the proportion of 10 to 90 per cent of the main oil, e.g. sweet almond.

Grapeseed oil

Note

Grapeseed is inexpensive compared to other oils.

Grapeseed oil originated in France but is now mainly produced in Spain, Italy and California. The plant is a climbing vine that produces grapes. The seeds of the grape yield a high quality oil that is almost colourless.

Uses of grapeseed oil

- Moisturising to the skin.
- Useful for clients who do not like oils that are too greasy.

Jojoba (ho-ho-ba) oil

Jojoba is a light yellow, waxy vegetable oil extracted from the crushed seeds of the jojoba shrub. This evergreen shrub grows in deserts and is native to Mexico, Arizona and California. It is a nutritious oil containing vitamin E, minerals and proteins, which are absorbed into the skin. Unlike many other oils, it can be heated to high temperatures and will still retain its nutrients.

At room temperature it is semi-solid due to its waxy consistency but solidifies when put in the fridge. It does not oxidise (mix with oxygen), therefore it keeps very well. It is good for all hair and skin types including oily skins.

Uses of jojoba

- Good for moisturising the skin.
- Helps to relieve inflammation so is excellent for acne, eczema, psoriasis and arthritis.
- Beneficial for all types of skin.

Jojoba is an expensive oil, so it is wise to use a small amount and mix it with another oil such as sweet almond. It is generally a safe oil to use.

Olive oil

Olive oil is a yellow/green oil extracted from the flesh of the olive. Olives are fruits grown on trees mainly in the Mediterranean. The oil has a thick consistency and strong odour so is often mixed with a lighter oil such as sweet almond. It is a good source of vitamin E and is useful for dehydrated and inflamed skin. It is an oil commonly used when cooking. It is preferable to use virgin or extra virgin oil.

Uses of olive oil

- Helps to moisturise the skin.
- Helps to relieve muscular stiffness and pain.
- Olive oil is a safe oil to use on the skin and rarely causes irritation; it is therefore an ideal oil to use on children.

Sunflower oil

The sunflower originated in South America, although it is now grown in many countries. The flower head produces seeds. Sunflower oil is obtained from these seeds. The oil contains vitamins A, D and E, and minerals including calcium and iron.

Uses of sunflower oil

◆ Beneficial for skin complaints and bruises.

◆ Thought to be helpful for leg ulcers.

◆ Often used in preparations for acne and skin disorders in which there is dryness and inflammation as it is softening and moisturising to the skin.

Wheatgerm oil

Note

Ensure the client is not allergic to wheat flour prior to using.

A cereal grass that is native to West Asia but also grown in other subtropical climates. The wheat grain at the top of the stem consists of the husk (bran), which surrounds the germ. The oil is extracted from the germ. The unrefined wheatgerm oil has a strong odour, which many people find unpleasant, so can be mixed with other oils.

Wheatgerm oil contains high levels of vitamin E, which is a natural antioxidant (prevents oxidation), so can be added to other oils to act as a preservative. The oil also contains vitamins A, B and many minerals.

Uses of wheatgerm oil

◆ Moisturises dry skins.

◆ Relieves symptoms of dermatitis.

◆ Beneficial for tired muscles and useful after exercise.

◆ It is good on ageing skin due to its natural antioxidants, helping to prevent oxidation of the cells, which causes the skin to wrinkle and age.

◆ It is softening to the skin and acts as a cell regenerator thus improving the condition of the skin.

Note

Although oxygen is essential to life it is also responsible for the deterioration (oxidation) of cells, such as skin cells. Antioxidants can help slow down this deterioration as they help prevent oxidation of the cells occurring.

Massage creams

Creams are softening to the skin and are useful for dry skin. They often have a pleasant aroma, making the massage more enjoyable. Creams absorb more readily than oils so may have to be reapplied more frequently. They can sometimes feel sticky when massaging.

Note

Remember to use a spatula when removing cream from a pot, as bacteria can enter the pot and contaminate the cream if fingers are used.

Talc/powders

Swedish massage was traditionally performed with talc as it helps to prevent sliding of the hands over the body so allows deeper pressure; therefore it is useful if carrying out sports massage in which deep massage movements are used. Cornflour or arrowroot may be preferred because the particles do not irritate the respiratory passages in the same way as talc. It is also thought that talc is carcinogenic (cancer causing substance), but some baby powders are now talcum free. Powder is useful to use on oily skin or on clients who do not like residues of oils or creams. However, it needs to be frequently applied during the massage treatment.

Note

On hairy surfaces some therapists prefer to use cream and some prefer to use powder. Practise on a hairy client and see which medium you prefer!

Mediums can be wiped off the body using eau-de-cologne according to the preference of the client.

To complete Table 4.4, research the information regarding massage mediums and briefly discuss the advantages and disadvantages of using them.

Table 4.4 Advantages and disadvantages of massage mediums

Medium	Brief description, include advantages and disadvantages
Oil	
Massage creams	
Talc/powders	

PRE-HEAT TREATMENTS

The effects of massage can be improved if the tissues are warmed before the treatment begins. The warmth causes the blood vessels to dilate and so increases the circulation, relieving pain and tension and helping induce relaxation.

There are a variety of pre-heat treatments including infra-red, paraffin wax, sauna and steam bath. All of these methods produce similar effects, but some are more suitable for heating specific areas such as joints, while others are used for warming the whole body.

Uses and benefits of heat treatments

- Promotes relaxation.
- Stimulates the blood circulation, thus increasing

oxygen and nutrients to the tissues and removing waste products.

- Increases lymphatic flow so speeds up the release of toxins.
- Relaxes muscles in preparation for massage.
- Relieves joint pain, tension and muscle spasm.
- Used before sport to warm the tissues so that flexibility is improved and the contractability of muscles is enhanced.
- Used after injury to aid healing and recovery. However, heat treatment should not be given for the first 72 hours after injury.

Infra-red treatment

Infra-red treatment can be used to treat localised areas such as muscle joints and the upper or lower back. Infra-red rays are electromagnetic waves and are given off from the sun and also any hot object, e.g. electric fires and gas fires. A special lamp is used to supply infra-red rays, which produce heat in the epidermis only. The heat is carried to the deeper tissues by the blood circulation.

Contra-indications to infra-red

- Skin that is hypersensitive or lacks sensitivity.
- Heart conditions and blood pressure disorders.
- Thrombosis or phlebitis.
- Bronchitis, asthma, hay fever or heavy colds and fevers.
- Headaches or migraines.
- Skin infections and disorders such as eczema or psoriasis.
- Diabetes.
- Epilepsy.
- Metal pins/plates.

- ◆ After a heavy meal.
- ◆ Later stages of pregnancy.
- ◆ First one or two days of period especially if heavy.
- ◆ Sunburn.

Treatment procedure

Ensure all manufacturers' instructions and precautions are followed so that injury does not occur. All electrical equipment must be fully checked before each use.

1 Switch on the lamp to warm it up. Ensure it faces away from the client and from the therapist's eyes.

2 Make sure that the area to be treated is clean and free of grease.

3 Areas of the body you do not wish to treat should be covered with towels. The client's eyes should be protected from the rays.

4 Position the lamp at a right angle to the body and place the lamp at a distance of 45–90 centimetres.

5 The area can be warmed for about 15 minutes (never perform massage under the infra-red lamp).

6 At the end of the treatment switch the lamp off and place it safely away from the client.

Paraffin wax

When paraffin wax is cold it is solid but when heated it becomes liquid. It is heated in a thermostatically controlled container and applied to the body using a brush. This treatment is particularly beneficial for arthritis sufferers as it helps ease stiffness in arthritic joints.

Note

Always check with insurers to see if they cover heat treatments, or whether further training is required.

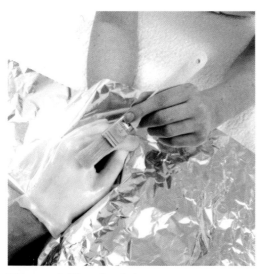

Figure 4.22a *Applying paraffin wax to the treatment area*

Contra-indications to paraffin wax

- Skin diseases and disorders.
- Cuts and bruises.

Treatment procedure

1 Apply a moisturising cream to the area.

2 Test the temperature of the paraffin wax by placing a small amount on the back of your wrist, then test the temperature on the client in the same way.

3 Using a bowl and brush, build up about five layers to the area.

4 Cover the treated area with tin foil and towels to keep in the heat.

5 Remove the wax when it has cooled by peeling it off and then continue with the massage.

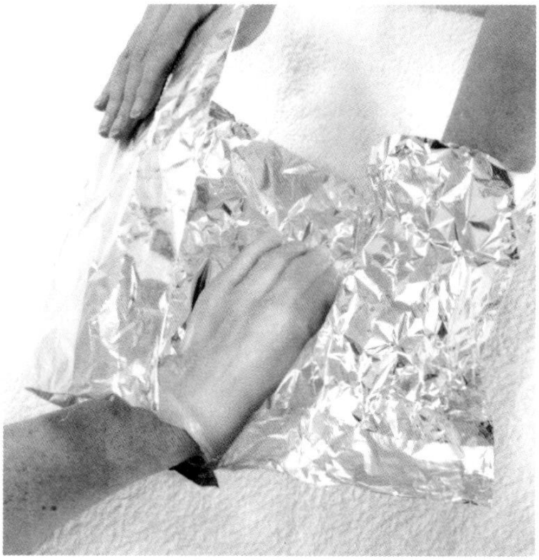

Figure 4.22b *Wrapping the area in foil*

Sauna bath

The heat produced in a sauna bath is a dry heat, not a moist heat as in a steam bath. Saunas are mostly made of logs with insulating material between them to prevent heat loss. The heat is produced from an electric stove, which is controlled by a thermostat.

To produce more heat, water can be poured on to coals using ladles. Treatment time is between 15 and 20 minutes and the client should be advised to have regular cool showers during the treatment and just prior to the massage.

Contra-indications to both steam and sauna baths

- Heart conditions.
- High/low blood pressure.
- Thrombosis.
- Skin diseases and disorders.

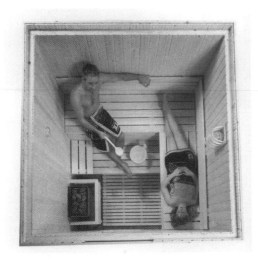

Figure 4.23 *Sauna bath*

- Epilepsy.
- Diabetes.
- Chest conditions, asthma and bronchitis.
- Pregnancy.
- Heavy menstruation.
- After a heavy meal or drinking alcohol.

Steam bath

A steam bath produces a moist heat as water is heated to produce steam. Steam baths are often made of fibreglass and have a door with an opening for the client's head. There is a seat with a tank underneath it, in which the water is heated producing wet steam. Treatment time is usually about 15 minutes and the client should shower prior to the massage treatment.

Task 4.4

Tick the relevant box that applies to each pre-heat treatment.

Table 4.5 Properties of pre-heat treatments

Heat treatment	Uses special lamp	Creates a dry heat	Used to warm specific areas of the body	Liquefies when warm and applied with a brush	Creates a moist heat	Can be used for generalised body warming
Infra-red						
Paraffin wax						
Sauna						
Steam bath						

1. Name **3** factors that influence an individual's posture.

....

....

....

2. Name and describe **3** postural faults.

....

....

....

3. Name the **2** working postures.

....

....

....

4. List the **4** main types of massage techniques.

....

....

....

....

5. List **3** types of medium used in massage.

....

....

....

6. Name and discuss **3** different types of oils used for massage treatment.

....

....

....

....

....

....

7. Briefly describe how you carry out a patch test to see if a client was allergic to an oil.

....

....

....

....

....

8. Name and briefly describe **4** types of pre-heat treatment.

....

....

....

....

....

....

....

PALPATION

An important part of massage is having the ability to know how soft tissues, such as muscle, should feel to the touch. Palpation is the art of feeling or sensing changes in the tissues and is incorporated into the massage routine. The fingertips are ideal to palpate the tissues as they contain numerous nerve receptors. They can detect temperature changes, different textures, and hardness and softness in tissues. Erythema may also be an indication of tension within a muscle.

If there is tension or maybe damage to the muscle tissue, the affected area will feel different. Sometimes the affected areas can be fairly large and easily felt by the client. Sometimes the problem can stem from a few damaged muscle fibres no thicker than a human hair. The client will probably feel discomfort when the affected area is touched and non-verbal communication such as teeth clenching will be an indication that there is a problem.

If the tissues feel normal when palpated but the client feels discomfort, work on the other side of the body and compare. If only one side is uncomfortable there may be a problem to treat so additional massage may be required.

Note

When palpating deeply into the tissues ensure that the thumb/fingers are supported by the thumb/fingers of the other hand to add some weight. This will help support the joints and minimise pressure on them.

This exercise will help you develop your palpating skills.

Cut about 4 centimetres of thread from a cotton reel and place a piece of paper over the top. Try to feel the piece of thread. Now place two pieces of paper on top and again try to feel the thread. Continue to place sheets of paper on top until the thread cannot be felt any more. This task will help develop your sense of touch.

THE ARRIVAL OF THE CLIENT

The trolley and couch should be prepared before the client arrives. If the client is an existing one check his or her record card to ensure there are no special requirements or any medical details that you need to be aware of. If the last time you both met you noted that the client was going on holiday perhaps this time you could ask if he or she enjoyed their holiday in France! Clients will feel you have an interest in them and what they are doing.

Note

Jewellery such as necklaces and earrings should be removed from the client prior to the massage to prevent it accidentally being broken. This will help to ensure the massage flows correctly.

FULL BODY MASSAGE

A full body massage will take about an hour, not including the consultation. When giving a body massage it is usual to begin on the front of the legs and complete the massage routine on the back. Generally, the head and face are not massaged as part of the routine.

The body parts may be massaged in the following order, although many routines will start with the back and shoulders instead.

1   Left leg (5 minutes)

2   Right leg (5 minutes)

3   Right arm (5 minutes)

4   Left arm (5 minutes)

5   Chest (5 minutes)

6   Abdomen (5 minutes)

Turn the client over.

7   Right leg (5 minutes)

8   Left leg (5 minutes)

9   Back (20 minutes)

These timings and order of work are guidelines only. If you or your client does not like a particular massage movement it can be left out. If a client requires particular attention to be paid to an area, e.g. the upper back, you may decide to spend 25–30 minutes on the back instead and so shorten the time spent massaging other areas.

It is important to adopt the correct posture when carrying out a massage. Always keep the back straight and the shoulders relaxed. When carrying out some of the massage movements ensure you bend your knees rather than bending at the waist; this will help to prevent strain and injury to your back.

Note

Most clients seem to prefer a deep massage but if the area is bony or tissues are thin use only light pressure.

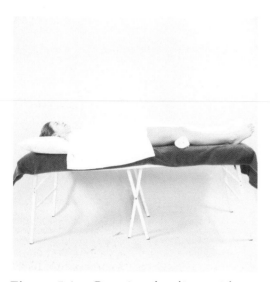

Figure 5.1 *Covering the client with towels*

During the massage contact should ideally be maintained at all times. If the therapist needs to reach something from the trolley one hand should remain in gentle contact with the client. If the trolley is on wheels it can be pulled towards you easily.

Clients can lay their head on a pillow and their body should be fully covered by towels as soon as they lie down. Two towels can be used: one large towel placed lengthways from the waist to feet and another placed across the chest between the neck and waist. As each body part is worked the area is uncovered and re-covered as the massage continues. When the client rolls over, the towel may be held down at one side so that the body continually remains covered. Blankets can be placed over the towel if the client feels cold.

Cushions can be used to support parts of the body. When the client is lying on his or her back (supine) a pillow or bolster can be placed under the knees and will help to flatten the lumbar region of the spine. This knee support is particularly useful for those clients with back pain.

When the client is lying on his or her front (prone) a cushion can be placed under the abdomen. This will help to round out the lumbar spine, making it more comfortable for clients with lordosis.

A tightly rolled towel can be placed under the ankles. This will prevent overstretching of the anterior tibial tendons and will shorten and relax the calf and hamstring muscles, and also prevent cramp occurring in the foot.

MASSAGE ROUTINE

Firstly clean the feet with surgical spirit or toner, such as rose water. Begin the massage on the front of the left leg.

Effleurage to sides and front of the leg (walk standing)

Place the whole hands flatly on to the ankle; the fingers and thumbs of each hand should be close together. Massage up and over the lower leg to the top of the thigh using the whole surface of the hands. Lightly stroke the hands down the sides of the legs and finish off the movement by sliding one hand over the front of the foot and the other underneath the foot, therefore sandwiching the foot. Hold the hands here for a few seconds. Repeat the whole movement four times.

Single handed kneading to the thigh (walk standing)

Place both hands on to the thigh, just above the knee, the fingers pointing towards the client's head. Use the palm of the hand nearest to the outer thigh to create circular movements to the outer thigh. Work gently upwards towards the top of the thigh. Swap hands, so that the other hand works on the front and inside of the thigh in an upward direction. Repeat the whole movement four times.

Double handed picking up to the thigh (stride standing)

Place both hands side by side on the thigh, about 5 centimetres apart, so that the fingers are

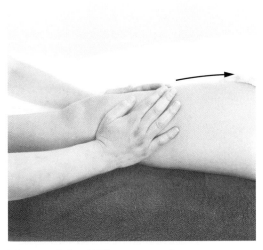

Figure 5.2 *Effleurage to leg*

> **Note**
>
> Ensure you work lightly over the inside of the thigh and bony areas.

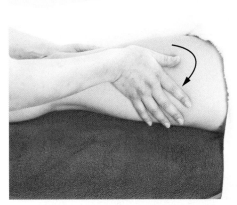

Figure 5.3 *Single handed kneading to thigh*

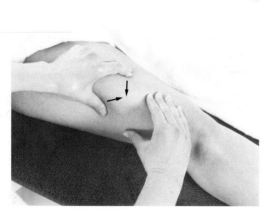

Figure 5.4 *Double handed picking up to the thigh*

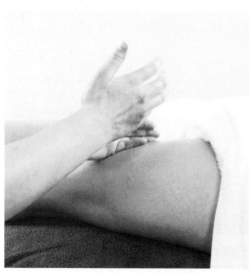

Figure 5.5 *Hacking to the thigh*

pointing towards the side of the couch. Create C shapes with the hands. Using one hand only, slide the fingers and thumb towards each other, and pick up and squeeze the tissues. As this hand releases the tissues, the other hand now lifts, squeezes and releases the tissues. The hands work alternately so that the whole thigh is worked.

Hacking to the thigh (stride standing)

Place the little-finger side of the hands (ulnar border) on to the thigh, about 5 centimetres apart. Ensure the hands are slightly cupped in shape. Alternately strike the thigh using the side of the hands, including the little finger and ring finger. Work at a fast pace and ensure the pressure is not too heavy. Work over the whole front of the thigh.

Cupping to the thigh (stride standing)

Cup both hands, ensuring the fingers and thumbs are close together, so there are no gaps between them. Alternately strike the thigh with the hands producing hollow sounds. Only the pads of the fingers and bottom part of the palm will be in contact with the body. Work over the whole front of the thigh.

Wringing to the thigh (stride standing)

Create C shapes with both hands and place them on to the thigh, the left hand positioned slightly forward of the other hand. Gently grasp the tissues between the fingers and thumbs of both hands. Pull forward the fingers of the left hand and push forward the thumb of the right hand. Lift and squeeze the tissues until a S shape is created and then release. Now pull the fingers of the right hand forward and push the left thumb forward, squeeze and release the tissues. Repeat this movement, working over the whole thigh.

Deep effleurage to the thigh (walk standing)

Place both hands flat, side by side above the knee. As you massage in an upward direction towards the top of the thigh, use your body weight to apply deeper pressure. Ensure the hands maintain contact on the return stroke, although the pressure will be light. Repeat these movements until the whole upper thigh has been worked.

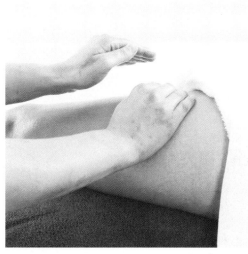

Figure 5.6   *Cupping to the thigh*

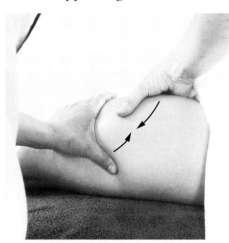

Figure 5.7a   *Wringing to leg*

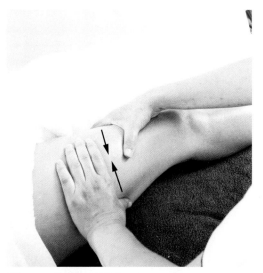

Figure 5.7b   *Wringing to leg*

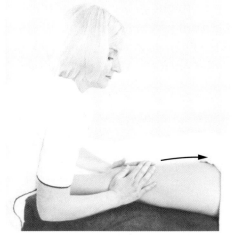

Figure 5.8   *Deep effleurage to thigh*

Note

Do not forget to link the massage movements together by using stroking or effleurage. Contact should be maintained at all times.

Thumb knead around patella (walk standing)

Place the pads of the thumbs at the top of the knee. Work around the patella creating small circular movements with the thumbs, working deep into the muscle. Work around the whole knee four times.

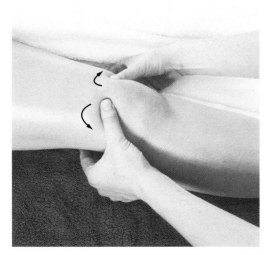

Figure 5.9 *Thumb knead around patella*

Effleurage to the lower leg (walk standing)

Place the whole hands flatly on to the ankle, ensuring the fingers and thumbs of each hand are close together. Massage over the lower leg towards the knee. Stroke the hands down the sides of the legs and finish off the stroke by sliding one hand over the front of the foot and the other underneath the foot. Hold the hands here for a few seconds. Repeat the whole movement four times.

Thumb knead to tibialis anterior muscle (walk standing)

One hand acts as a support on the inner side of the lower leg and the other hand is positioned just below the knee. The thumb is used to create small, circular movements to the anterior tibial muscle, working from just below the knee towards the ankle. Then stroke the hand back up towards the starting position. Repeat the whole movement twice.

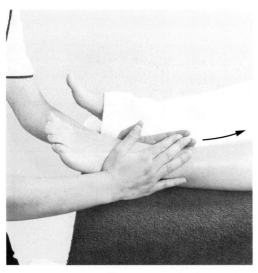

Figure 5.10 *Effleurage to the lower leg*

Finger knead around bones of ankle (stride standing)

Place the hands on either side of the ankle. Use the pads of the fingers to create small, circular movements around the joint of the ankle. Repeat this movement four times.

Thumb stroke to dorsal surface of foot (stride standing)

Holding on to the foot with both hands, fingers positioned underneath each side of the foot and the thumbs placed just above the toes. Stroke the thumbs upwards and over the dorsal surface of the foot, working especially between the tendons of the foot. Stroke the whole area four times.

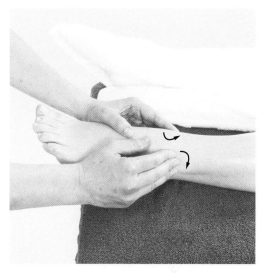

Figure 5.12 *Finger knead around bones of ankle*

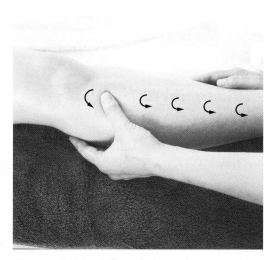

Figure 5.11 *Thumb knead to anterior tibial muscle*

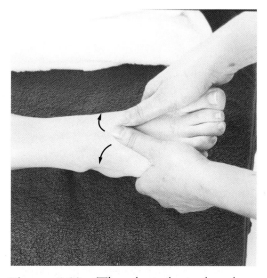

Figure 5.13 *Thumb stroke to dorsal surface of foot*

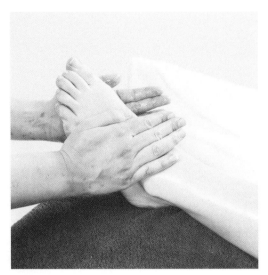

Figure 5.14 *Effleurage to bottom of foot*

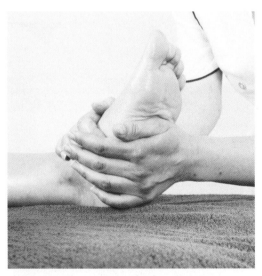

Figure 5.15 *Palmar knead to bottom of foot*

Effleurage to bottom of foot (walk standing)

Place one hand on the dorsal surface of the foot and use the palm of the other hand to effleurage from the top to the bottom of the plantar surface of the foot. Repeat four times.

Palmar knead to bottom of foot (walk standing)

Place one hand on the dorsal surface of the foot to support and the other hand on the plantar surface of the foot. Use the palm of this hand to make circular movements, ensuring the whole bottom of the foot is worked.

Thumb stroke to bottom of foot (zig-zag) (stride standing)

Place the fingers of both hands on the dorsal surface of the foot. Position the thumbs on the bottom of the foot below the toes. Alternately stroke across the foot with the thumbs, in a zig-zag motion. Repeat this movement until the whole bottom of the foot has been worked.

Note

If the pressure is too light this movement may tickle the client.

Circular thumb knead to bottom of foot (stride standing)

Place the fingers on the dorsal aspect of the foot and the thumbs just beneath the toes. Use the pads of the thumbs to perform small, circular movements. Work over the whole of the bottom of the foot.

Effleurage to bottom of foot (walk standing)

Place one hand on the dorsal surface of the foot and use the palm of the other hand to effleurage the plantar surface of the foot, from the top to the bottom of the foot. Repeat four times.

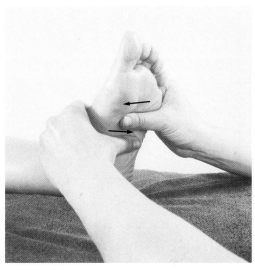

Figure 5.16 *Thumb stroke to bottom of foot*

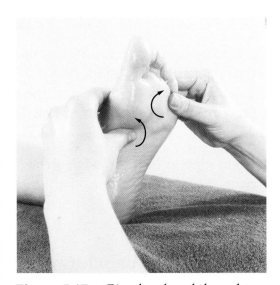

Figure 5.17 *Circular thumb knead to bottom of foot*

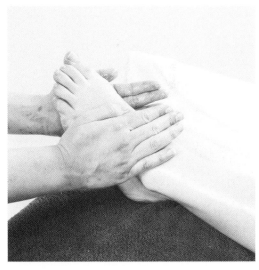

Figure 5.18 *Effleurage to bottom of foot and whole leg*

Repeat this whole sequence on the right leg.

Complete Table 5.1 by stating which bones and muscles are worked over during each massage movement. See Chapter 2 for a reminder of the relevant anatomy and physiology.

Table 5.1 Massage movements and bones and muscles worked over

Massage movement	Name of bone or bones worked over	Name of muscle or muscles worked over
Single handed kneading to thigh		
Effleurage to lower leg		
Palmar knead to bottom of foot		

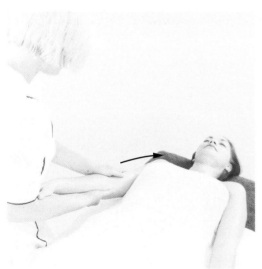

Figure 5.19 *Effleurage to outside of whole arm*

Now move on to massaging the arms. Begin the massage on the right arm.

Effleurage to outside of whole arm (walk standing)

Use one hand to support the arm and the other hand to massage. Effleurage over the outer lower and upper arm. Use light pressure to stroke back down the arm. Repeat this movement four times.

Thumb knead to triceps muscle (walk standing)

Use one hand to support the arm and the other hand to massage. Use the pads of the thumbs to create circular movements over the triceps muscle. Work over the whole back of the upper arm.

Single handed picking up to triceps muscle (walk standing)

Use one hand to support the arm and the other hand to massage. Use the fingers and thumb to pick up, squeeze and lift the triceps muscle. Release the tissues and continue working over the whole back of the upper arm.

Thumb knead to outer forearm (walk standing)

Use one hand to support the arm and the other to massage. Use the pad of the thumb to create small, circular movements to the outer forearm. Work over the whole outer forearm.

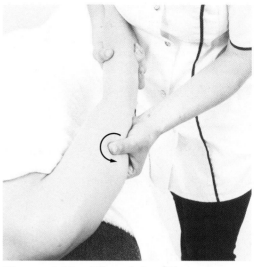

Figure 5.20 *Thumb knead to triceps muscle*

Note

Ensure you do not massage over bony areas.

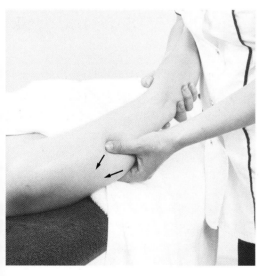

Figure 5.21 *Single handed picking up to triceps muscle*

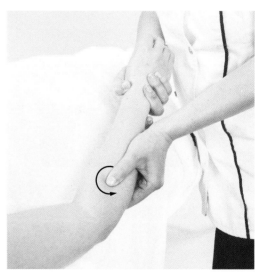

Figure 5.22 *Thumb knead to outer forearm*

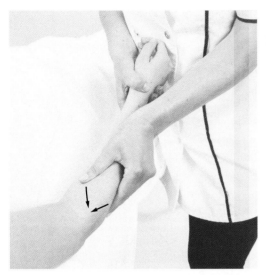

Figure 5.23 *Single handed picking up to outer forearm*

Single handed picking up to outer forearm (walk standing)

Use one hand to support the arm and the other to massage. Use the fingers and thumb to pick up, lift and squeeze the tissues. Release the tissues and continue to work over the whole outer forearm.

Effleurage to whole of inside arm (walk standing)

Use one hand to support the arm and the other hand to massage. Effleurage over the whole inside of the arm. Use light pressure to stroke back down the arm. Repeat this movement four times.

Thumb knead to biceps muscle (walk standing)

Use one hand to support the arm and the other to massage. Use the pad of the thumb to create small, circular movements to the inside upper arm. (The fingers can rest on the back of the arm.) Work over the whole area.

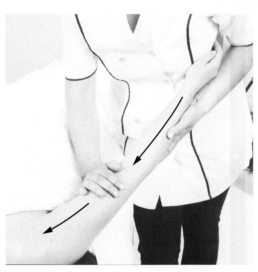

Figure 5.24 *Effleurage to whole of inside arm*

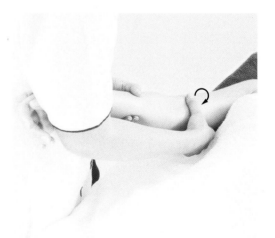

Figure 5.25 *Thumb knead to biceps muscle*

Pick up to biceps muscle (walk standing)

Use one hand to support the arm and the other hand to massage. Use the fingers and thumb to squeeze and lift the biceps muscle. Release the tissues and continue working over the whole inside of the upper arm.

Thumb knead to inner forearm (walk standing)

Use one hand to support the arm and the other hand to massage. Use the pad of the thumb to create circular movements over the inner forearm. Work over the whole area.

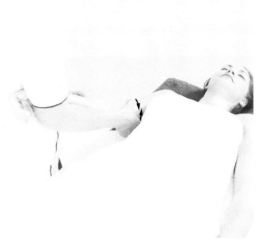

Figure 5.26 *Pick up to biceps muscle*

Pick up to inner forearm (walk standing)

Use one hand to support the arm and the other to massage. Use the fingers and thumb to pick up, lift and squeeze the tissues. Release the tissues and continue to work over the whole inner forearm.

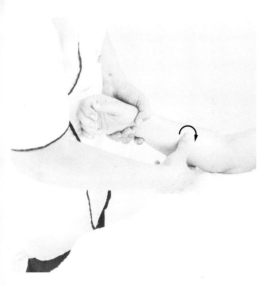

Figure 5.27 *Thumb knead to inner forearm*

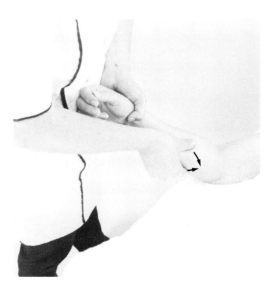

Figure 5.28 *Pick up to inner forearm*

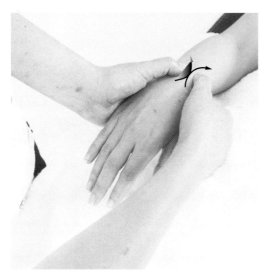

Figure 5.29 *Thumb knead around wrist joint*

Thumb knead around wrist joint (walk standing)

Place both thumbs on to the wrist. Use the pads of the thumbs to create small, circular movements around the joints of the wrists. Repeat this movement four times.

Thumb stroking to back of hand (walk standing)

Hold the client's hand firmly with both hands. Use the thumbs to stroke between the tendons of the hands. Continue to stroke over the whole back of the hand.

Circular thumb knead to joints of fingers and thumbs (walk standing)

Hold the client's hand firmly with one hand. Use the pad of the thumb of the other hand to make small, circular movements to all the joints of the fingers and thumb.

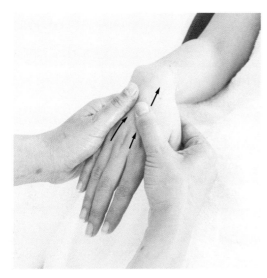

Figure 5.30 *Thumb stroking to back of hand*

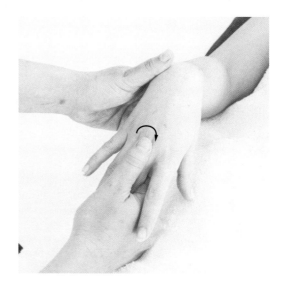

Figure 5.31 *Circular thumb knead to joints of fingers and thumbs*

Thumb stroking to palm of hand (walk standing)

Hold the client's hand firmly with one hand, the palm facing upwards. Use the pad of the thumb of the other hand to stroke the palm of the client's hand. Ensure the whole palm is worked.

Circular thumb kneading to palm of hand (walk standing)

Hold the client's hand firmly with one hand. Use the pad of the thumb of the other hand to create small circles on the palm of the client's hand. Ensure the whole palm is worked.

Effleurage to outside and inside of whole arm (walk standing)

Use one hand to support the arm and the other hand to massage. Effleurage over the whole outside of the arm. Use light pressure when stroking back down the arm. Repeat this movement four times. Then repeat this movement to the inside of the whole arm.

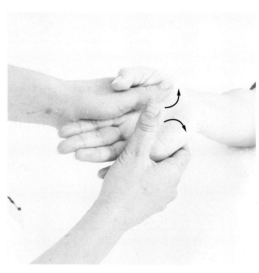

Figure 5.32 *Thumb stroking to palm of hand*

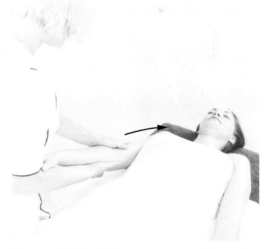

Figure 5.34 *Effleurage to outside and inside of whole arm*

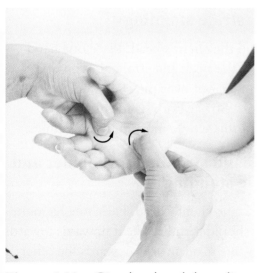

Figure 5.33 *Circular thumb kneading to palm of hand*

Repeat this whole sequence on the left arm.

Complete Table 5.2 by stating which bones and muscles are worked over during each massage movement.

Table 5.2 Massage movements and bones and muscles worked over

Massage movement	Name of bone or bones worked over	Name of muscle or muscles worked over
Effleurage to inside of upper arm		
Single handed kneading to outer forearm		
Thumb knead to inner forearm		
Circular thumb kneading to palm of hand		
Effleurage to outside of upper arm		

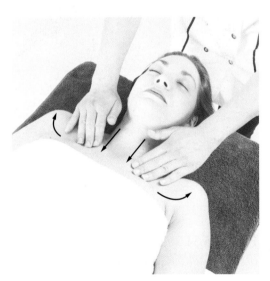

Figure 5.35 *Effleurage to sides of neck, chest and shoulders*

Now, move on to chest massage.

Effleurage to sides of neck, chest and shoulders (stride standing)

Stand behind the client's head. Place one hand either side of the neck and stroke down both sides. Effleurage out over the chest and around the shoulders. Stroke both hands back to the neck. Repeat this whole movement four times.

Alternate hand stroking to shoulder and neck (stride standing)

Stand behind the client's head. Place one hand on to the right shoulder and stroke it upwards towards the neck. As one hand strokes upwards the other hand is placed on to the right shoulder and strokes upwards. Alternately stroke the right shoulder and neck with the hands. Repeat movement four times and then massage the left side.

Knuckling to chest (stride standing)

Stand behind the client's head. Create loose fists with your hands, the fingers and knuckles slightly apart. Make circular movements with the fingers, using the parts of the fingers about 2.5 centimetres down from the nail to massage the whole chest area. Press lightly over bony areas and avoid working directly on the breasts if massaging a woman.

Finger and thumb kneading to muscles of chest and upper back (stride standing)

Stand behind the client's head. Place the fingers on each shoulder and use the pads of the fingers to create small, circular movements over the chest and then use the pads of the thumbs to create small, circular movements over the trapezius muscle.

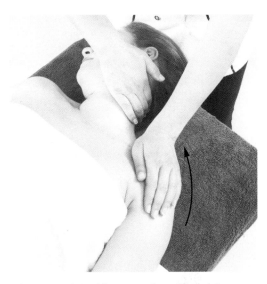

Figure 5.36 *Alternate hand stroking to shoulder and neck*

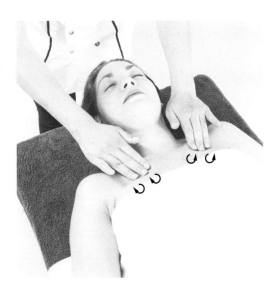

Figure 5.38 *Finger and thumb kneading to muscles of chest and upper back*

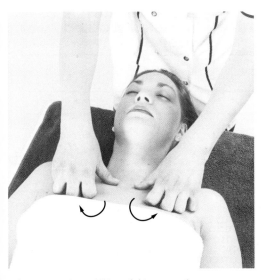

Figure 5.37 *Knuckling to chest*

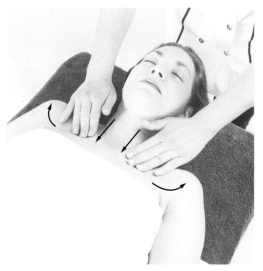

Effleurage to sides of neck, chest and shoulders (stride standing)

Stand behind the client's head. Place one hand either side of the neck. Stroke down either side of the neck and effleurage over the chest and out over the shoulders, then stroke the fingers back to the neck. Repeat this movement four times.

Figure 5.39 *Effleurage to sides of neck, chest and shoulders*

Task 5.4

Complete Table 5.3 by stating which bones and muscles are worked over during each massage movement.

Table 5.3 Massage movements and bones and muscles worked over

Massage movement	Name of bone or bones worked over	Name of muscle or muscles worked over
Alternate hand stroking to shoulder and neck		
Knuckling to chest		
Thumb kneading to muscles of upper back		

Now move on to the abdomen. Always massage in a clockwise direction on the abdomen, following the direction of the colon.

Clockwise stroking to abdomen (stride standing)

Stand to the side of the couch. Use alternate hands to stroke in a clockwise direction around the abdomen. Repeat this movement four times.

Finger kneading to abdomen (stride standing)

Place one hand on top of the other and create small circles with the fingers. Work in a clockwise direction around the abdomen ensuring the pressure used is light. Repeat this movement four times.

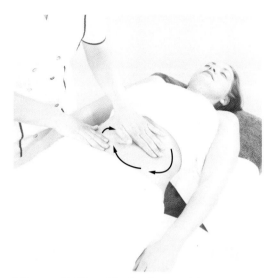

Figure 5.40 *Clockwise stroking to abdomen*

Wringing to waist (stride standing)

Create C shapes with both hands and place them on to the side of the waist furthest from you, the left hand positioned slightly forward of the other hand. Gently grasp the tissues between the fingers and thumbs of both hands. Pull forward the fingers of the left hand and push forward the thumb of the right hand. Lift and squeeze the tissues to create a S shape and then release. Now pull the fingers of the right hand forward and push the left thumb forward, squeeze and release the tissues. Work up and down the side of the waist. Repeat the whole movement to the other side of the waist.

Skin rolling to waist (stride standing)

Begin on the side of the waist furthest from you. Create C shapes with both hands and press the fingers on to the skin of the waist, using the thumbs to push and roll the flesh towards the fingers. Release the movement and move the

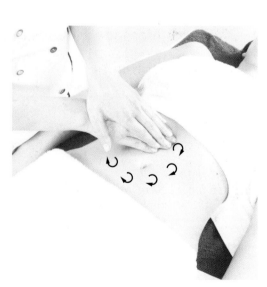

Figure 5.41 *Finger kneading to abdomen*

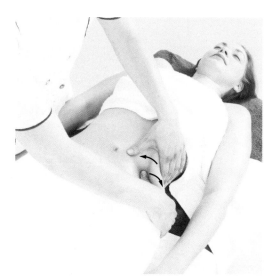

Figure 5.42 *Wringing to waist*

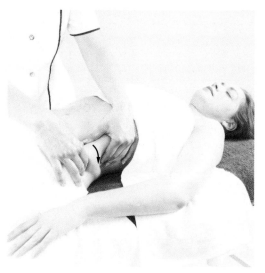

Figure 5.43 *Skin rolling to waist*

hands to work on another area until the whole side of the waist has been worked. Standing in the same position repeat this movement on the side of the waist nearest to you.

> **Note**
>
> Wringing and skin rolling can be left out if there is little tissue present around the waist.

Alternate hand stroking to waist (stride standing)

Begin on the side of the waist furthest from you. Use the hands to alternately stroke in an upward direction working over the sides of the waist. Standing in the same position, repeat this movement on the other side of the waist, turn the palms to face upwards and stroke the hands in an upward direction on the waist.

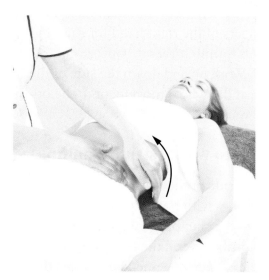

Figure 5.44 *Alternate hand stroking to waist*

Effleurage to abdomen (walk standing)

Position the hands side by side on the abdomen above the pubis. Slide the hands upwards until the fingers reach the bottom of the sternum. Slide the hands down either side of the waist and then return to the starting position. Repeat this movement four times.

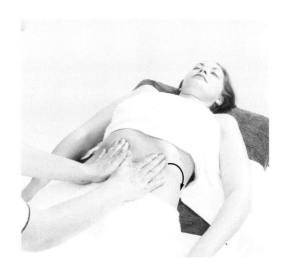

Figure 5.45 *Effleurage to abdomen*

Task 5.5

Complete Table 5.4 by stating which bones and muscles are worked over during each massage movement.

Table 5.4 Massage movements and bones and muscles worked over

Massage movement	Name of bone or bones worked over	Name of muscle or muscles worked over
Alternate hand stroking to waist	*None*	
Effleurage to abdomen	*None*	

Turn the client over; remember to ensure the client is fully covered by the towels as they roll over. Begin the massage on the back of the right leg. A pillow can be placed under the abdomen and bolsters under the ankles if required.

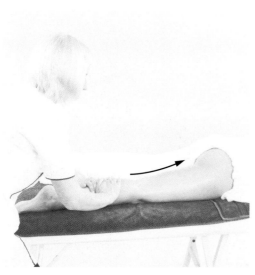

Figure 5.46 *Effleurage to whole leg and buttock*

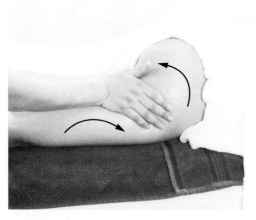

Figure 5.47 *Single handed kneading to thigh and buttock*

Effleurage to whole leg and buttock (walk standing)

Place both hands on to the ankle; the fingers and thumbs of each hand should be close together. Use the whole surface of the hands to massage over the lower leg, thigh and over the buttock. Stroke the hands down the sides of the legs and finish off by sliding both hands over the bottom of the foot. Repeat the whole movement four times.

Single handed kneading to thigh and buttock (walk standing)

Place both hands on to the thigh, just above the knee. One hand rests on the thigh for support. Use the palm of the other hand to create circular movements over the thigh. Work upwards towards the top of the thigh and over the buttock, then stroke back to the starting position. Swap hands, so that the other hand massages another area of the thigh, working in an upward direction.

Double handed picking up to thigh (stride standing)

Place both hands side by side on the thigh so that fingers point to the side of the couch, about 5 centimetres apart. Make C shapes with the hands. Using one hand only, slide the fingers and thumb towards each other so that the tissues are picked up and squeezed. As one hand releases the tissues, the other hand now lifts, squeezes and releases the tissues. The hands work alternately up and down the thigh so that the whole thigh is worked over.

Hacking to the thigh and buttock (stride standing)

Place the little-finger side of the hands (ulnar border) on to the thigh, about 5 centimetres apart. Ensure the hands are slightly cupped in shape. Alternately strike the thigh using the side of the hands including the little finger and ring finger. Work at a fast pace and ensure the pressure is not too heavy. Work over the back of the thigh and buttock.

Beating to thigh and buttock (stride standing)

Loosely clench both fists, backs of the hands facing upwards. With loose wrists alternately strike the area using fairly deep pressure. Work over the whole back of the thigh and over the buttock area.

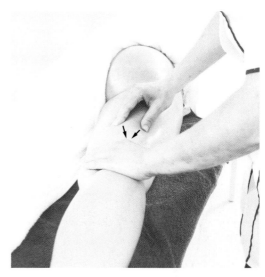

Figure 5.48   *Double handed picking up to thigh*

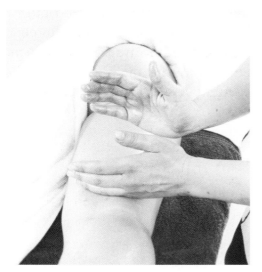

Figure 5.49   *Hacking to the thigh and buttock*

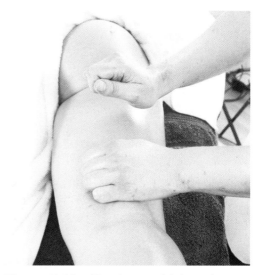

Figure 5.50   *Beating to thigh and buttock*

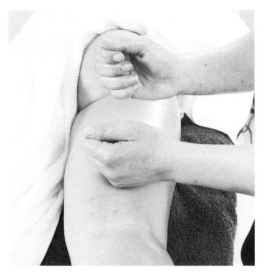

Figure 5.51 *Pounding to thigh and buttock*

Pounding to thigh and buttock (stride standing)

Loosely clench both fists and position the hands so that the thumbnails face upwards. Abduct the elbows. The area is struck using the little-finger side of the hands (ulnar border). As one fist strikes the body the other fist lifts off. The fists circle each other, alternately pounding the skin. Work over the thigh and buttock.

Wringing to thigh (stride standing)

Create C shapes with both hands and place them on to the thigh, the left hand positioned slightly forward of the other hand. Gently grasp the tissues between the fingers and thumbs of both hands. Pull forward the fingers of the left hand and push forward the thumb of the right hand. Lift and squeeze the tissues to create a S shape and then release. Now pull the fingers of the right hand forwards and push the left thumb forwards, squeeze and release the tissues. Repeat this movement, ensuring the whole back of the thigh is worked.

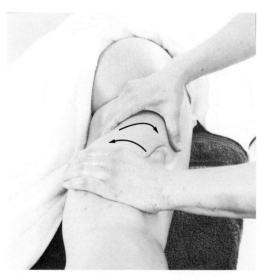

Figure 5.52 *Wringing to thigh*

Effleurage to whole back of leg (walk standing)

Place both hands on to the ankle; the fingers and thumbs should be close together. Massage over the lower leg to the top of the thigh using the whole of the hands. Stroke the hands down the sides of the legs and finish off the stroke by sliding both hands over the bottom of the foot. Repeat the whole movement four times.

Single handed kneading to lower leg (walk standing)

Rest one hand on the lower leg and use the other palm to create circular movements over the calf. Work in an upwards direction towards the back of the knee. Ensure the whole back of the lower leg is worked.

Double handed picking up to lower leg (stride standing)

Place both hands side by side on the calf so that fingers point towards the side of the couch, about

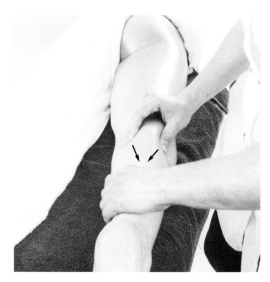

Figure 5.53 *Effleurage to whole back of leg*

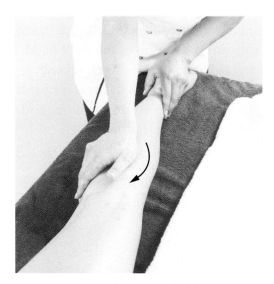

Figure 5.54 *Single handed kneading to lower leg*

Figure 5.55 *Double handed picking up to lower leg*

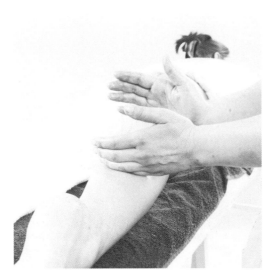

Figure 5.56 *Hacking to lower leg*

5 centimetres apart. Make C shapes with the hands. Using one hand only, slide the fingers and thumb towards each other so that the tissues are picked up and squeezed. As one hand releases the tissues, the other hand now lifts, squeezes and releases the tissues. The hands work alternately up and down the back of the lower leg so that the whole area is worked.

Hacking to lower leg (stride standing)

Place the little-finger side of the hands (ulnar border) on to the back of the lower leg, about 5 centimetres apart. Ensure the hands are slightly cupped in shape. Alternately strike the calf using the side of the hands including the little finger and ring finger. Work at a fast pace and ensure the pressure is not too heavy. Work up and down the lower leg.

Wringing to lower leg (stride standing)

Create C shapes with both hands and place them on to the calf, the left hand positioned slightly forward of the other hand. Gently grasp the tissues between the fingers and thumbs of both hands. Pull forward the fingers of the left hand and push forward the thumb of the right hand. Lift and squeeze the tissues and then release. Now pull the fingers of the right hand forwards and push the left thumb forwards, squeeze and release the tissues. Repeat this movement, ensuring the whole back of the lower leg is worked.

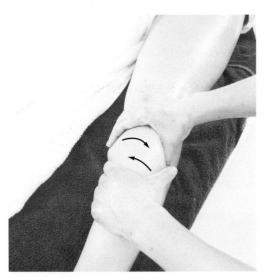

Figure 5.57 *Wringing to lower leg*

Effleurage to whole leg and buttock (walk standing)

Place both hands on to the ankle, the fingers and thumbs of each hand close together. Massage over the lower leg, the top of the thigh and over the buttock using the whole surface of the hands. Stroke the hands down the sides of the legs and finish off the stroke by sliding both hands over the bottom of the foot. Repeat the whole movement four times.

Now massage the back of the left leg.

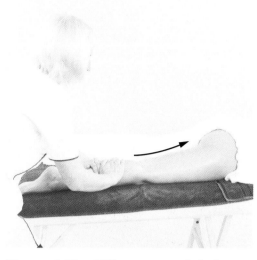

Figure 5.58 *Effleurage to whole leg and buttock*

Task 5.6

Complete Table 5.5 by stating which bones and muscles are worked over during each massage movement.

Table 5.5 Massage movements and bones and muscles worked over

Massage movement	Name of bone or bones worked over	Name of muscle or muscles worked over
Double handed picking up to thigh		
Hacking to lower leg		

Now, move on to massaging the back.

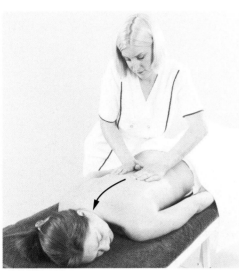

Figure 5.59 *Effleurage to back*

Effleurage to back (walk standing)

Place both hands at the base of the back, either side of the spine, pointing towards the head. Keep the hands flat and slide them forwards, working up either side of the spine, towards the neck. Stroke the hands down either side of the back returning to the starting position. Repeat this movement four times, ensuring the whole back is massaged.

Single handed kneading to back (walk standing)

Rest one hand on the left side of the lower back and use the other palm to create circular movements to the right side of the back. Work up the back and massage over the shoulder. Continue working over the whole right side of the back. Swap hands and knead the left side of the back.

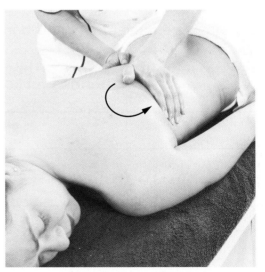

Figure 5.60 *Single handed kneading to back*

Reinforced palmar kneading around scapulae (walk standing)

Place one hand on to the shoulder, fingers pointing towards the head, and lay the other hand on top to reinforce the movement. Work around the scapula and over the shoulder, applying pressure with the fingers and palms to fleshy areas and easing off pressure over bony areas. Repeat this movement four times and then work on the other shoulder.

Circular thumb knead to shoulders (walk standing)

Place your left hand on the left shoulder and your right hand on the right shoulder. Use the pads of the thumbs to perform small, circular movements to the muscles of the upper back. Work over the whole upper back, avoiding any bony areas.

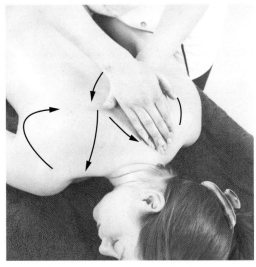

Figure 5.61   *Reinforced palmar kneading around scapulae*

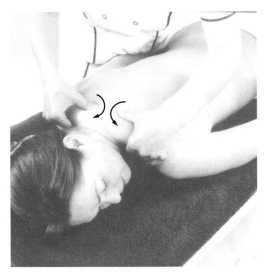

Figure 5.62   *Circular thumb knead to shoulders*

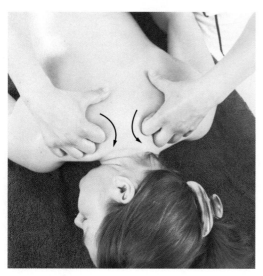

Figure 5.63 *Knuckling to back*

Knuckling to back (walk standing)

Make loose fists with your hands, the fingers and knuckles slightly apart. Place the hands on to the back and create circular movements with the fingers, using the parts of the fingers about 2.5 centimetres down from the nail to massage the area. Massage the whole of the back, taking care not to apply too much pressure over the kidneys and to avoid bony areas.

Effleurage towards lymph nodes (walk standing)

Place both hands at the base of the back, pointing towards the head. Keeping the hands flat slide the hands forwards, either side of the spine, up towards the neck. Push the fingers over each shoulder. Stroke the hands back down to the base of the back and then slide the hands forward

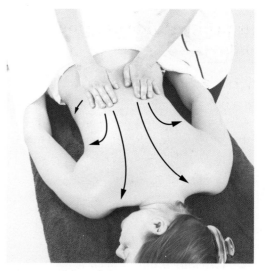

Figure 5.64 *Effleurage towards lymph nodes*

towards the underarm (axillary) areas. Stroke the hands back to the base of the back and slide the hands over the waist towards the abdominal area. Stroke the hands back to the starting position. Repeat this whole movement four times.

Thumb kneading/frictions to either side of spine (walk standing)

Place the thumbs at the base of the back, either side of the spine, just above the sacrum. Use the pads of the thumbs to create small, circular movements and work up the back, either side of the spine towards the neck. Stroke the hands down the back returning to the starting position. Repeat the movement four times.

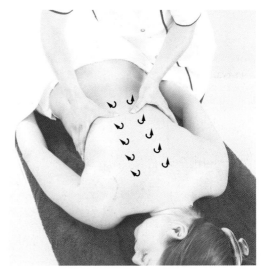

Figure 5.65 *Thumb kneading/frictions to either side of spine*

Note

If there are any knots, perform the frictions movements to help disperse them. See Chapter 4 for the correct techniques.

Vibrations to either side of spine (walk standing)

Place the knuckles of the index and middle fingers of one hand at the base of the neck, either side of the spine. The other hand can be placed on the shoulder. Vibrate the knuckles so that a tremor is produced. Work down either side of the spine towards the base of the back. Repeat the whole movement twice.

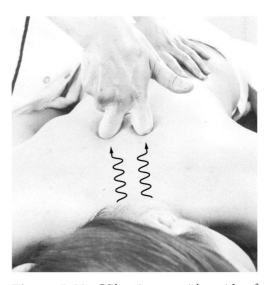

Figure 5.66 *Vibrations to either side of spine*

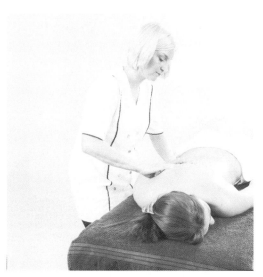

Figure 5.67 *Double handed picking up to back*

Double handed picking up to back (stride standing)

Place both hands side by side on the back, about 5 centimetres apart, so that fingers point to the side of the couch. Make C shapes with the hands. Using one hand only, slide the fingers and thumb towards each other so that the tissues are picked up and squeezed. As one hand releases the tissues, the other hand now lifts, squeezes and releases the tissues. The hands work alternately up and down the back and over the shoulder area so that the whole back is worked.

Skin rolling to waist and hips (stride standing)

Create C shapes with both hands and press the fingers on to the right side of the back, using the thumbs to push and roll the flesh towards the fingers. Release the movement and move the hands to work on another area. When the whole area has been worked over, remain in the same position and repeat the movement on the other side of the back.

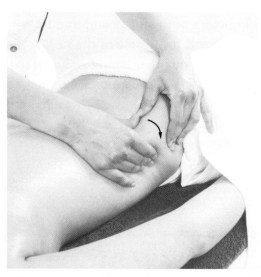

Figure 5.68 *Skin rolling to waist and hips*

Palmar knead to lower back (walk standing)

Place one hand on the lower back to support and the other hand at the base of the back. Use the palm of this hand to make circular movements, ensuring the whole lower back is worked. Use both hands alternately if necessary. Use only light pressure over the kidney areas.

Thumb knead to lower back (walk standing)

Place both hands on to the lower back. Use the pads of the thumbs to perform small, circular movements to the muscles of the lower back. Work over whole lower back, including around the sacrum. Avoid the kidneys and any bony areas.

Light hacking to whole back (stride standing)

Place the little-finger side of the hands (ulnar border) on to the back, about 5 centimetres apart. Ensure the hands are slightly cupped in shape.

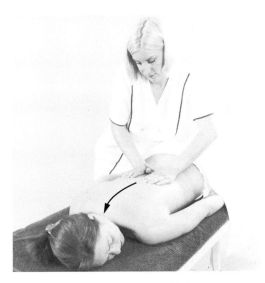

Figure 5.69 *Palmar kneading to lower back*

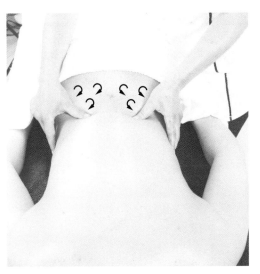

Figure 5.70 *Thumb knead to lower back*

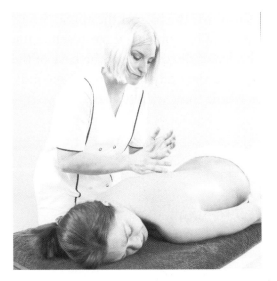

Figure 5.71 *Light hacking to whole back*

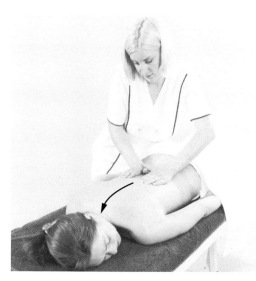

Figure 5.72 *Effleurage to whole back*

Alternately strike the back using the side of the hands including the little finger and ring finger. Avoid any bony areas. Work at a fast pace and ensure the pressure is not too heavy. Work up and down the whole back.

Effleurage to whole back (walk standing)

Place both hands at the base of the back, pointing towards the head. Keeping the hands flat, slide them forwards, either side of the spine, up to the neck. Stroke the hands back down to the base of the back. Repeat the whole movement four times.

Cover the client's back with a towel and, before leaving the client to rest for a while, carry out a spinal stretch.

Spinal stretch and rocking over towel (stride standing)

Place both hands side by side on the middle of the spine, so they are pointing towards the side of the couch. Slide both hands slowly sideways so that one hand works towards the neck and the other slides towards the base of the spine. Stretch along the spine. When one hand has reached the top of the back and the other is at the base of the back, gently rock the body for about six seconds. Repeat this whole movement twice.

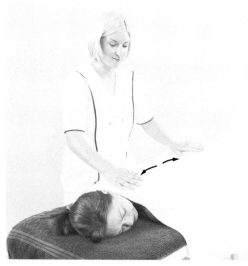

Figure 5.73 *Spinal stretch and rocking over towel*

Note

It is advised to allow the client to rest for about 5 to 10 minutes after the massage treatment.

Complete Table 5.6 by stating which bones and muscles are worked over during each massage movement.

Table 5.6 Massage movements and bones and muscles worked over

Massage movement	Name of bone or bones worked over	Name of muscle or muscles worked over
Circular knead to shoulders		
Thumb knead to sides of spine		
Double handed picking up to back		
Skin rolling to sides of back		
Palmar knead to lower back		

BODY MASSAGE ROUTINE AT A GLANCE

Try to complete a full body massage within an hour.

Front of leg massage

Begin on the left leg.

- Effleurage to sides and front of the leg (walk standing).
- Single handed kneading to the thigh (walk standing).
- Double handed picking up to the thigh (stride standing).
- Hacking to the thigh (stride standing).
- Cupping to the thigh (stride standing).
- Wringing to the thigh (stride standing).
- Deep effleurage to the thigh (walk standing).
- Thumb knead around patella (walk standing).

> **Note**
>
> When practising the routine put this book into a transparent plastic bag to prevent staining the pages with oil.

- Effleurage to lower leg (walk standing).
- Thumb knead to tibialis anterior muscle (walk standing).
- Finger kneading around bones of ankle (stride standing).
- Thumb stroke to dorsal surface of foot (stride standing).
- Effleurage to bottom of foot (walk standing).
- Palmar knead to bottom of foot (walk standing).
- Thumb stroke to bottom of foot (zig-zag) (stride standing).
- Circular thumb kneading to bottom of foot (stride standing).
- Effleurage to bottom of foot and whole leg (walk standing).
- Effleurage to bottom of foot and whole leg (walk standing).

Repeat this whole sequence on the right leg.

Arm massage

Begin the massage on the right arm.

- Effleurage to outside of whole arm (walk standing).
- Thumb knead to triceps muscle (walk standing).
- Single handed picking up to triceps muscle (walk standing).
- Thumb knead to outer forearm (walk standing).
- Single handed picking up to outer forearm (walk standing).
- Effleurage to whole of inside arm (walk standing).
- Thumb knead to biceps muscle (walk standing).
- Pick up to biceps muscle (walk standing).
- Thumb knead to inner forearm (walk standing).
- Pick up to inner forearm (walk standing).
- Thumb knead around wrist joint (walk standing).
- Thumb stroking to back of the hand (walk standing).

- Circular thumb knead to joints of fingers and thumbs (walk standing).

- Thumb stroking to palm of hand (walk standing).

- Circular thumb kneading to palm of hand (walk standing).

- Effleurage to whole inside and outside of arm (walk standing).

Repeat this whole sequence on the left arm.

Chest massage

- Effleurage to sides of neck, chest and shoulders (stride standing).

- Alternate hand stroking to shoulders and neck (stride standing).

- Knuckling to chest (stride standing).

- Finger and thumb kneading to chest and upper back muscles (stride standing).

- Effleurage to sides of neck, chest and shoulders (stride standing).

Abdomen massage

- Clockwise stroking to abdomen (stride standing).

- Finger kneading to abdomen (stride standing).

- Wringing to waist (stride standing).

- Skin rolling to waist (stride standing).

- Alternate hand stroking to waist (stride standing).

- Effleurage to abdomen (walk standing).

Turn client over. Begin on the back of the right leg.

Back of leg massage

- Effleurage to whole leg and buttock (walk standing).

- Single handed kneading to thigh and buttock (walk standing).

- Double handed picking up to thigh (stride standing).

- Hacking to thigh and buttock (stride standing).
- Beating to thigh and buttock (stride standing).
- Pounding to thigh and buttock (stride standing).
- Wringing to thigh (stride standing).
- Effleurage to whole leg (walk standing).
- Single handed kneading to lower leg (walk standing).
- Double handed picking up to lower leg (stride standing).
- Hacking to lower leg (stride standing).
- Wringing to calf (stride standing).
- Effleurage to whole leg and buttock (walk standing).

Now massage the back of the left leg.

Back massage

- Effleurage to back (walk standing).
- Single handed kneading to back (walk standing).
- Reinforced palmar kneading around scapulae (walk standing).
- Circular thumb knead to shoulders (walk standing).
- Knuckling to back (walk standing).
- Effleurage towards lymph nodes (walk standing).
- Thumb kneading/frictions to either side of spine (walk standing).
- Vibrations to either side of spine (walk standing).
- Double handed picking up to back (stride standing).
- Skin rolling to waist and hips (stride standing).
- Palmar knead to lower back (walk standing).
- Thumb kneading to lower back (walk standing).
- Light hacking to whole back (stride standing).
- Effleurage to whole back (walk standing).
- Spinal stretch and rocking (stride standing).

Note

Using 'stroking' movements at the end of the massage is very soothing.

CONTRA-ACTIONS, ALSO KNOWN AS HEALING CRISIS

After a massage treatment the client will usually feel relaxed and reap the benefits of the treatment, but occasionally a client may experience a contra-action. A contra-action is a reaction that may happen during or after the massage treatment.

During treatment the following contra-action may occur:

- Erythema is reddening of the skin and often indicates that the massage is reaching the deeper layers of the skin, therefore increasing nutrition and encouraging removal of waste products from the area.

- A client may experience aching or soreness in the muscles, due to the release of toxins and the body's nerves responding to the deep massage work.

- The release of toxins may also cause tiredness. The body will need to rest to enable its healing energies to carry out their work effectively. After the tiredness has disappeared the client should feel refreshed and full of energy!

- The client may feel a little emotional, perhaps even tearful. It can be a good way for the client to release tension.

After treatment

Occasionally a client may report any of the following reactions up to 24–48 hours after treatment.

- headache
- nausea
- thirst
- sleepiness
- frequent urination.

Many of these contra-actions will be due to the flushing out of toxins and will soon settle down.

Note

Ensure you note any contra-actions that may occur.

AFTERCARE ADVICE

After the treatment the client should be given the following aftercare advice so that he or she gains maximum benefit from the treatment. The aftercare advice should be followed for 24 hours.

- Rest and relax. Encourage client to practise deep breathing and relaxation techniques. This will help ensure that the body is able to heal itself sufficiently.

- Drink lots of water to help flush out toxins from the body.

- Avoid sunbathing or sunbed treatments unless all of the oil is removed in case the skin burns.

- Eat only small meals. Eating large meals will cause blood to be diverted to the gut to help with the digestion of food. The demands of digestion will divert energy away from the healing processes. Light meals such as fruit and vegetables make ideal snacks.

- Avoid coffee, tea and colas as they contain caffeine. Caffeine is a stimulant and therefore will not help the client to relax.

- Do not smoke or drink alcohol for about 24 hours as the treatment is a detoxifying one and smoking and drinking will introduce toxins into the body.

As part of the aftercare advice postural and mobility exercises may be given if necessary. You could design a leaflet that would include these exercises and also relaxation and breathing techniques. Advice regarding stress and how to deal with its negative effects may also be useful to the client.

Study the information given on aftercare advice opposite to enable you to answer the questions listed here.

1 What should a client drink after treatment and why?

. . . .

. . . .

2 Why should a client eat only small meals after treatment?

. . . .

. . . .

3 Why should a client avoid alcohol consumption and smoking after treatment?

. . . .

. . . .

4 Why should a client be encouraged to relax after treatment?

. . . .

. . . .

5 Why should sunbathing or sunbed treatments be avoided after massage?

. . . .

. . . .

6 In what drinks would you find caffeine? Why should caffeine be avoided after a treatment?

. . . .

. . . .

CASE STUDY GUIDELINES

You may be required to carry out case studies as part of your course. The following guidelines will help you write up the information.

Consultation

Carry out a consultation using a consultation form and write a summary to include the following:

- Information about client's lifestyle and any health considerations, e.g. varicose veins.
- What are the client's expectations, e.g. to alleviate aches and pains, help to relax, etc?
- Write a treatment plan for the client.

Massage treatment and aftercare advice

> **Note**
>
> See Chapter 6 for discussion of postural and mobility exercises.

- Did you use specific massage movements – perhaps there were tension nodules?
- Name any particular muscle you worked on specifically – maybe you found knots or tension within it.
- Did the client enjoy certain massage movements more than others?
- Did you have to change the massage treatment in any way – perhaps your client is elderly and you could only massage certain areas of the body?
- Did the client suffer with fluid retention, so were specific lymphatic drainage massage movements used?
- What aftercare advice did you give?
- Were there any postural faults – did you give postural exercises?
- Was there stiffness in the joints – did you give mobility exercises?
- Did you recommend breathing or relaxation exercises?

Effectiveness of the treatment

- Was the treatment effective? How did your client feel?
- Were there any contra-actions?
- Do you think you could have improved the treatment? If so, what would you have done differently?
- What positive or negative comments did your client make after the treatment?
- Ask the client to fill out a client feedback form to find out what he or she thought of the treatment.

Next treatment

- When the client visits you again ask he or she how they felt after the last treatment.
- Was the treatment beneficial?
- Did he or she experience any contra-actions?
- Has the client's health altered in any way?
- Have you made any changes to the treatment plan?

Summary

On the final treatment write a conclusion summing up all of the treatments and how effective they were and how you dealt with any problems.

Case Study

Emily Snadden is 24 years old, single and has no children. She works as a primary schoolteacher and although she enjoys her job she finds it very stressful. She has a healthy lifestyle with frequent exercise and eats regular nutritious meals. She also drinks lots of water. She does not smoke and drinks little alcohol.

Emily complains of a stiff neck and tense shoulders. She also suffers with lower backache. She would like a relaxing massage.

I observed her posture and noticed her back was hollow and abdomen was protruding (lordosis). She has no contra-indications.

Client name   *Ms E. Snadden*   **Date of treatment**   *31st January 2003*
Treatment given   *Body massage*

What are the client's expectations of treatment?
To be relaxed.
To ease tension in the neck and shoulders.
To ease lower backache.

What are the treatment objectives?
To use lots of effleurage massage movements and avoid the use of tapotement movements so that the massage is relaxing.
To use petrissage movements such as kneading, wringing and knuckling to ease the tense muscles. Use frictions movements to help treat knots within muscles.
To pay attention to the lower back using petrissage movements to help ease lower backache.

Oil chosen and amount used:
Grapeseed (25 ml)

Any special needs? *(e.g. help on to couch, the client is pregnant, etc)*
Client has lordosis so placed a pillow under the abdomen to help round out the lumbar region.

Recommended frequency of treatment *Client will return for treatment once a week for 6 weeks.*

Additional notes:
I have recommended specific postural exercises and given advice on how to correct posture to help with lordosis.
I advised a mobility exercise for her neck.
I have given relaxation and breathing exercises that will help her cope with stressful situations.

Figure 5.74 *Treatment plan for Ms Snadden*

Treatment one

A full body massage was given but particular attention was paid to her back and neck. As the client has lordosis, when she was lying on her front I placed a cushion under her abdomen to help round out the lumbar region of the spine, so that she was more comfortable.

I used mostly kneading and knuckling massage movements to work deep into the trapezius muscle to help relieve tension. I found two knots within the trapezius muscle, so used frictions movement to help disperse them. I used thumb kneading on the neck area, working either side of the spine to help ease the stiffness in the neck. I avoided the use of tapotement movements to ensure the massage was relaxing.

I gave her aftercare advice and leaflets informing her how to carry out the postural and mobility exercises safely. I also gave advice and a leaflet explaining the breathing and relaxation techniques to help her deal more effectively with stress.

Treatment two

Emily said she slept well after the first treatment and definitely felt relief from the tension in her neck and back. She has been practising the postural and mobility exercises regularly and found the relaxation techniques particularly useful.

During this treatment I paid most attention to the back and neck. I worked on knots I found within the trapezius muscle. I also worked on the lower back using lots of kneading movements. In addition Emily had some fluid retention around the ankles. She had had a long day and been standing for long periods of time. I elevated the legs and used lymphatic drainage movements to help disperse the fluid.

I explained it was important to follow aftercare advice to gain the full benefit of the treatment.

Treatment three

Emily had had a particularly stressful week and had used the breathing and relaxation exercises a great deal. She said she was still suffering from tension in her shoulders. However, the lower backache had much improved and this was no longer causing her pain.

As usual I paid most attention to the shoulder and neck areas. The muscles felt hard and tense, and it was a little uncomfortable for her, so I applied lighter pressure than before and noticed that there was a lot of erythema, perhaps indicating there was tension in that area. I used plenty of effleurage movements in between the petrissage movements to help soothe and relax the muscles.

Treatment four

Emily said she had great relief from the last treatment although she did feel a little nauseous afterwards. I explained this may be due to the release of toxins that had built up.

I told her it was important that she tried to relax her shoulders as much as possible to avoid them becoming tense. I informed her that tension in the shoulders may lead to headaches.

Summary

I feel Emily benefited a great deal from the treatments and she said she really enjoyed them and would return for more treatments. She regularly carries out the postural and mobility exercises and felt these had helped her. She uses the breathing and relaxation exercises daily, especially at work.

The stiffness in her neck has eased and her lower backache has much improved. I feel she will need more treatments to help with the tension in her shoulders though. The knots were hard to disperse and obviously require more work.

I took far too long on the first treatment and felt very
nervous but my confidence has grown lots since then, and
by the fourth treatment the massage took an hour to
perform.

1. Why are the muscle tissues palpated during massage treatment?

   . . . .

   . . . .

   . . . .

2. Why would you check a client's medical details every time they
   came for treatment?

   . . . .

   . . . .

   . . . .

3. Why should jewellery be removed from the client prior to massage
   treatment?

   . . . .

   . . . .

   . . . .

4. How would you position the towels on your client?

   . . . .

   . . . .

   . . . .

5. Discuss how cushions or bolsters can be used as support for the client during massage treatment.

. . . .

. . . .

. . . .

6. What precautions would you take to avoid cross-infection?

. . . .

. . . .

. . . .

7. Discuss the contra-actions that may occur during treatment.

. . . .

. . . .

. . . .

8. How long would a full body massage (including consultation) normally take?

. . . .

9. List **4** contra-actions that may happen 24–48 hours after treatment.

. . . .

. . . .

. . . .

10. State **3** pieces of aftercare advice you would give to the client.

. . . .

. . . .

. . . .

Considerations and Modifications to the Massage Treatment and Other Types of Physical Therapy

6

It is important that the massage treatment meets with the client's expectations and it may require modification in some way to suit the client's needs.

ADAPTING MASSAGE FOR SPECIFIC CONDITIONS

Relaxing massage

Many clients want massage treatment purely for relaxation. A relaxing massage will often include lots of effleurage, and little if any tapotement movements are used. Music may help the client to relax.

Poor muscle tone

Ageing and sedentary lifestyles with little exercise can cause the muscles to become flabby, with poor muscle tone. Tapotement and vibration movements are particularly useful to help stimulate muscle tone.

Oedema

Ensure the oedema is non-medical before proceeding with treatment. If there is fluid retention in the feet and ankles: with the client on the couch, raise the legs above the level of the groin. If the oedema is in hands and wrists: the hands are raised above the axillae (underarm areas). Massage movements that help drain lymph towards lymph nodes are particularly useful. Firstly effleurage the area, knead and then use the whole hand to squeeze up the whole length of the limb, working slowly section by section towards the lymph glands.

Obese client

These clients may require firmer pressure, but not necessarily, so get regular feedback while massaging. You may find these clients will take a little longer to massage. Unfortunately massage does not break down fat, although the look of the skin can be improved owing to the stimulation of the blood circulation. When working over fatty areas effleurage and petrissage movements can be firmer and brisker to stimulate the blood and lymphatic circulations. Stimulating movements such as tapotement should be included to help soften the areas of hard fat, and is particularly useful for clients on slimming diets and undertaking regular exercise.

Cellulite is a condition found mainly in women where areas of adipose tissue (fat) become hard and lumpy. The affected area looks dimpled and lumpy, similar to the appearance of orange peel and often feels cool to the touch. It is mainly found in overweight people but also affects slim individuals and those of ideal weight.

Cellulite is very difficult to break down and remove and there are many factors that contribute to its build-up, including the hormone oestrogen that triggers the laying down of fat. To help with this condition a client should be advised to eat a low-fat diet, drink around 2 litres of water each day and take plenty of exercise. Regular massage treatment can help increase the blood and lymphatic circulation and so aid the removal of toxins that often build up in these areas due to poor circulation. Poor circulation occurs because the overloaded fat cells compress the blood and lymphatic capillaries.

Male clients

Men have tougher, thicker skin than women and are generally hairier. The subcutaneous layer often contains little fat and so there is easier access to the muscle tissue. Men often prefer a deep massage, so the therapist can use the body weight to add depth. The following factors should be taken into account when treating a man.

- Do not work too close to the groin area. It is advised not to massage the lower stomach and the inner thigh area.

- If the body is hairy, oil or powder are the best mediums to use and will probably need to be reapplied regularly.

- Work in the direction of the hair growth to help avoid discomfort due to pulling of the hairs.

Elderly or very slim clients

Elderly or very slim clients will probably prefer lighter pressure during massage treatment. Massage lightly over bony areas to avoid discomfort. If muscle tone is poor care must be taken when performing petrissage and tapotement movements, as they may be uncomfortable for the client. A hand or foot massage may be all that is possible for some elderly clients.

Treating minors and special needs clients

A minor refers to anyone under the age of 18 and minors should not be treated unless a parent or guardian is present, or has given written permission for treatment to take place. If a client is between 16 and 18 years old asking for parental permission may be contentious. If there are other people around it should be all right to carry out treatment but there should be caution if treating a person of the opposite sex.

Children and special needs clients respond very well to massage treatment. It is advised to carry out a relaxing massage using lots of effleurage and avoid using tapotement movements. A shorter time may be given for massage treatment.

If, while treating a minor or special needs client, he or she claims that abuse has taken place or you suspect there has been abuse, it is advisable to tell a superior.

Any unsuitable behaviour or signs of prior abuse should be noted. Any explanations given for these signs should be recorded and treated confidentially. The therapist must report any abnormal statement, event or observation to a senior person in the workplace.

Massage for clients with disabilities

It will depend on the severity of the disability as to what massage treatment can be given. The massage will need to be adapted to suit each individual. If a client uses a wheelchair, a hand and foot massage may be given. Generally the massage movements used will be mainly effleurage and petrissage. Tapotement movements should be avoided.

Pregnant clients

A pregnant client should check with her doctor or midwife before having massage treatment, as pregnancy can bring a variety of contra-indications such as high blood pressure. Pregnancy can be a stressful and tiring time for women, so massage can be particularly beneficial. The legs and feet can become particularly tired, especially as the weight increases and there may be fluid retention around the ankles. There can be difficulty with sleeping so the relaxing effects of massage are very useful. The body massage can be adjusted in the following ways:

- Use plenty of effleurage movements and avoid tapotement movements.

- Lie the client on her side with pillows under the arm and thigh so that you can massage the back and back of the legs. Alternatively the client can sit on a chair with a pillow on her lap.

- When she is lying on her back put a small pillow under the knees to relax the abdomen and flatten the lower back. Ensure the back of the couch is slightly raised as some pregnant women may feel faint and nauseous when lying flat on a couch.

- After the first trimester (three months) gentle stroking and effleurage massage movements may be performed on the abdomen.

Back massage for pregnant clients

If the client would like a back massage treatment she can sit by the side of the couch on a low-backed chair. Turn the chair around so that you can easily access the back and she can sit astride the chair with a large, soft cushion or pillow to fully support the abdomen. Pillows are placed on to the couch so the client may rest her head and arms on to it.

The therapist can kneel down on one knee, ideally with support under the knee.

Suggested back massage routine for pregnant women
(Look at Chapter 5 again to familiarise yourself with the following massage movements.)

1 Effleurage to back.

2 Single handed kneading to back.

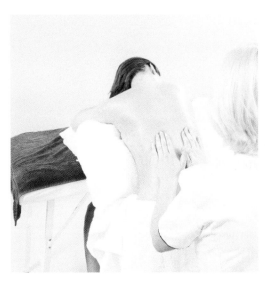

Figure 6.1 *Massage on a pregnant client*

3 Reinforced palmar kneading around scapulae.

4 Circular thumb kneading and picking up to shoulders.

5 Knuckling to back.

6 Effleurage towards lymph nodes.

7 Thumb kneading either side of spine.

8 Vibrations either side of spine.

9 Palmar knead to lower back.

10 Thumb knead to lower back.

11 Light hacking to whole back.

12 Effleurage to whole back.

Clients unable to lie in the prone position (on their front)

Occasionally there may be a reason why clients cannot lie in the prone position. Perhaps they are pregnant or suffer with asthma. The client may be late so you have to shorten the body massage treatment time. Therefore you may want to treat the front and back of the legs without having to turn the client over.

You will need a bolster or rolled-up medium- to large-sized towel to place underneath the knees to create space under the legs so you can massage the backs of them.

Leg massage

1 Effleurage to the front and the back of both legs. You may wish to raise the knee so that it is easier to massage the back of the legs. Repeat four times.

2 Kneading with the palms to the front of the client's right thigh.

3 Double handed picking up to the right thigh.

4 Single handed picking up to the back of the right thigh.

5 Palmar knead to the back of the right thigh.

6 Stroking around the knee.

7 Thumb knead to tibialis anterior muscle.

8 Bend the knee and pick up to the back of the right calf.

9 Palmar knead to back of the right calf.

10 Now repeat steps 2–9 to the left leg.

11 Effleurage to front and back of legs.

Complete Table 6.1 by briefly describing each type of modification to massage.

Table 6.1 Modifications to massage

Modification to massage	Briefly describe how treatment is modified and any considerations when giving treatment
Relaxing massage	
Treating poor muscle tone	
Oedema	
Obese clients	
Male clients	
Elderly or very slim clients	
Treating minors and special needs clients	
Clients with disabilities	
Pregnant clients	
Clients unable to lie in prone position	

Massage and mobility exercises to treat stiffness in the joints

Providing there are no contra-indications, massage and mobility exercises can be given to joints that are stiff. The stiffness may cause some discomfort for the client.

The therapist can advise mobility exercises for the client to do at home. These exercises will help to loosen the joints and relieve contracted areas within muscles. Ensure the client is fully aware how to carry out the exercises safely and that there is no medical reason why the client cannot perform these exercises.

Neck mobility

The client may sit or stand.

1 With the chin tucked in, drop the head slowly forward and then lift it back to the starting position. Repeat the whole movement four times.

2 With the chin tucked in, turn the head to face the right shoulder and then turn the head to face the left shoulder. Repeat the whole movement four times.

Stiff shoulder joint

If the shoulder joint is stiff massage should be given to all the muscles that act on that shoulder joint. These include the muscles of the arm, neck, chest, back and whole shoulder girdle. Deep frictions and finger kneading can be applied to the area around the joint, followed by lots of effleurage.

Shoulder mobility exercise

The client may sit or stand.

1 Shrug the shoulders up and relax back down. Repeat four times.

2 Circle the shoulders forwards for five seconds. Circle the shoulders backwards for five seconds. Repeat four times.

Elbow joint

Massage should be given to the whole arm, although particular attention should be paid to the muscles directly above and below the joint. Frictions can be applied to area around the joint.

Elbow mobility exercise

1 Bend the arm at the elbow so that the fingers touch the shoulder, then straighten the arm. Repeat four times.

Wrist, hand and finger joints

Massage to the whole arm is given but with emphasis on the forearm and hand.

Wrist mobility exercise

1 Circle one hand clockwise and then anti-clockwise. Repeat four times on each hand.

2 Supinate and pronate the arm, so the hand turns to face upwards, then downwards. Repeat four times to each hand.

Trunk mobility

Ask clients to stand with arms by their sides and check their posture.

1 With the chin tucked in, bend the trunk to the right and then to the left. Repeat four times each side.

2 With the hands on the hips twist the trunk to the right and then to the left. Repeat four times to each side.

Hip joint

If the hip joint is stiff, the client can lie on his or her side with a pillow placed between the knees for comfort. This enables the therapist to massage the hip. Particular attention is paid to the buttock, thigh and lumbar region muscles.

Hip mobility exercises

The client will need to stand next to a wall for support.

1 Lift one leg and circle at the hip for five seconds. Repeat this movement with the other leg.

2 Lift one leg and gently swing it forwards, sideways and backwards. Repeat whole movement twice. Repeat on other leg.

Knee joint

Massage can be given to the whole leg, although particular attention is paid to the quadriceps. Deep friction can be applied around the knee joint with the knee in semi-flexion.

Knee mobility exercises

The client will need to stand next to a wall for support.

1 With one leg bent at the knee, gently lift the bent knee upwards, as if reaching to touch the chest. Then slowly straighten the leg. Repeat this movement four times and then work the other leg.

2 With one leg bent at the knee lift the lower leg backwards and upwards, then straighten the leg. Repeat four times and then work the other leg.

Ankle, foot and toe joints

Massage should be given to the muscles of the lower leg. Finger kneading and frictions can be performed to the anterior tibialis, around ankle joints, and into the muscles of the foot to help with joint stiffness.

Ankle mobility exercises

The client may stand or sit.

1 Circle one foot clockwise and then anti-clockwise. Repeat four times on each foot.

2 Pull the foot up (dorsi flex) and then down (plantar flex). Repeat four times on each foot.

Task 6.2

Research the mobility exercises given above to complete Table 6.2.

Table 6.2 Mobility exercises

Body part	Brief description of one mobility exercise
Neck	
Shoulder	
Elbow	
Wrist	
Trunk	
Hip joint	
Knee	
Ankle	

OTHER TYPES OF MASSAGE TECHNIQUES

It is advisable first to practise the basic massage routine and to undertake a professional course of study before attempting the following massage movements, many of which are advanced massage techniques.

Deep tissue massage

Deep tissue massage techniques include deep stroking, deep effleurage, deep petrissage and deep friction. They help to reduce muscular tension caused by shortened and contracted muscles. When muscles are shortened and tense the blood and lymph cannot flow freely through the muscles, resulting in a build-up of waste products.

To release contracted muscles, slow compressive strokes are applied along their length, from origin to insertion, covering the tendons and bellies of the muscles. Specific strokes are then used to treat smaller sections of the muscle that may be abnormal. These strokes may be applied along the length of the muscles, following the direction of the muscle fibres, or performed across them, and are also used on the tendons to help minimise scar tissue formation. When these strokes are used messages are sent through the nervous system to inform the muscle to lengthen and relax. Deep tissue strokes are also applied to adjacent muscles to help reduce adhesions, such as scar tissue build-up, and will also help prevent and release fascias adhering to each other, so muscles can move independently of each other.

Deeply contracted muscle fibres can be felt as knots or lumps in the belly of the muscle. The lumps feel like crystals or tiny grains and are usually uncomfortable to the touch. They are due to the build-up of waste products caused by fatigue, injury or overuse and respond well to deep finger pressure such as frictions massage movements. Knots or lumps may also indicate that scar tissue is forming and may be found in tendons too. Deep tissue massage helps to break up and eliminate scar tissue.

Muscles that are continually contracted hold the bones out of position, which may lead to postural problems. Ligaments are also put under strain as they try to keep joints in place. This makes the body more prone to injury as muscle fibres that cannot lengthen are more likely to be torn during quick and vigorous movement. Injury is mostly likely to occur where the muscle meets the tendon or where the tendon joins with the periosteum of the bone.

Most deep tissue massage techniques are intended to bring balance to the body by lengthening shortened and contracted muscle fibres and the fascia that surround them. Muscles act in pairs so when muscles contract the opposing muscle is stretched. Muscles that remain contracted will mean the antagonistic muscle will stay in a lengthened position, which may weaken it. Therefore, once the shortened muscles have been lengthened, the stretched muscles may be strengthened with specific exercises.

Deep tissue strokes

The deep tissue strokes are a combination of slow, compressive and lengthening massage movements that help to relax contracted muscles and break down knots.

Some examples of deep tissue strokes follow:

1 *Lengthening movements*
  The fingers, thumbs, knuckles, forearm or base of the palm can be used to perform slow, gliding compression movements working in the same direction as the muscle fibres, from origin to insertion. These movements help to relax contracted muscle.

2 Criss cross

Using the pad of the thumb, work on a section of muscle about 2 centimetres square. Perform up-and-down movements, working in the direction of the muscle fibres and then side-to-side movements, working across the muscle fibres. The fingers may also be used.

3 Thumb circles

Use the pads of the thumbs to create fairly deep and small circular movements to the area. The fingers may also be used.

4 Finger stroking

With the hands side by side, fingers together, stroke the fingers of the right hand over the skin, creating a fairly small circular movement in a clockwise direction. The left hand will also make a circular movement, although in an anti-clockwise direction. This stroke helps to stretch the fascia covering the muscle.

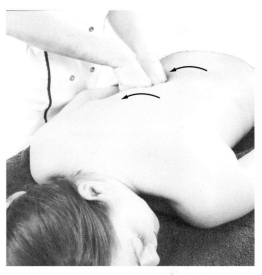

Figure 6.2 *Knuckles across latissimus dorsi muscle (lengthening movement)*

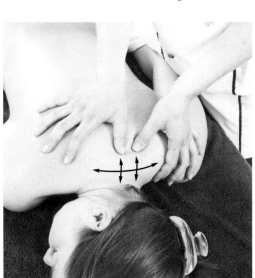

Figure 6.3 *Criss cross to trapezius*

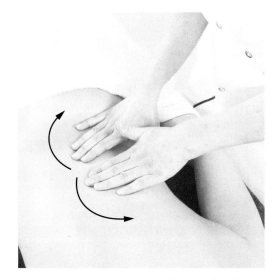

Figure 6.4 *Finger stroking to back*

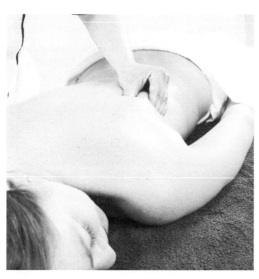

Figure 6.5 *Muscle rolling to back*

5 *Frictions*

First, stroke the area with the thumb. Place the thumb directly into the muscle tissue at a 90-degree angle to the surface of the body and use the other thumb and your body weight to lean into it. Apply deeper and deeper pressure into the tissues and then release. The fingers (the middle finger placed on top of the index finger), knuckles or elbows may also be used. This stroke is used on extremely contracted sections of muscle fibres.

6 *Muscle rolling*

Grasp a section of muscle tissue between the fingers and thumb. Roll the fibres to release any adhering of the muscle fibres. The sticking together of muscle fibres can be due to scar tissue or injury.

Neuromuscular techniques (NMT)

Neuromuscular (nerve-muscle) massage is a deep tissue massage technique developed in America. It consists of using deep friction techniques.

Muscular pain can be caused by injury, emotional stress, poor posture or overuse of muscles. Trigger points will be found in most cases and are small areas of hypersensitivity within muscles that form due to muscular strain. Sometimes several trigger points may be found clustered within the same muscle. The client will feel pain or discomfort when there is pressure applied at these points.

Neuromuscular massage treatment involves locating these trigger points. Deep massage strokes can be used to find them and the therapist will often feel areas of contraction in the affected muscle. It is thought that a trigger point is due to a restricted blood flow, therefore there is a build-up of waste products in the muscle fibres over a period of time. There is pressure placed on the nerves, which may radiate pain to other areas of the body, known as referred pain zones.

Neuromuscular techniques involve using the pads of the thumbs and/or fingers to apply deep and firm massage to the affected area. Neuromuscular massage uses different massage movements with the fingers and thumbs such as circling, four-finger stroking, pressures on a specific point, effleurage away from the spine and petrissage along nerve pathways. The arms are generally kept straight so that the therapist can use his or her body weight to add depth.

> **Note**
>
> At sites of trauma in the muscle, the surrounding muscle tissue will be contracted to help to protect it.

Treating a trigger point

1   First, use the pads of the index, middle and ring fingers (the thumbs, knuckles or elbow may also be used) to palpate and rub an area of muscle tissue about 3 centimetres square. The other hand can be used to lightly stretch the skin. Rub the area, working in an up-and-down movement, in the same direction as the muscle fibres. Then massage using a side-to-side movement, so that you are working across the muscle fibres. This will increase blood flow to the area resulting in erythema.

2   Work over the same area using the thumb or fingers slowly and deeply to stroke the skin. Ask the client to tell you when he or she feels any areas of discomfort or pain.

3   When a trigger point is located ask the client to breathe in and then apply deep pressure on to the area as he or she breathes out using the thumb (ensure the pad of one thumb is placed on top of the other to support it). Apply pressure directly to the trigger point for up to 90 seconds. Usually the pain will ease at about 30 seconds

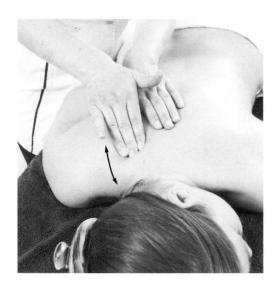

Figure 6.6 Rubbing area in preparation

so when the client no longer feels discomfort release the pressure and continue to work on another area. The area can be returned to a number of times during the massage treatment if needed.

Applying pressure to the trigger point disrupts the flow of nerve impulses that cause referred pain, so clearing the nerve pathways, therefore reducing

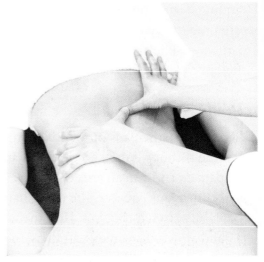

Figure 6.7a NMT

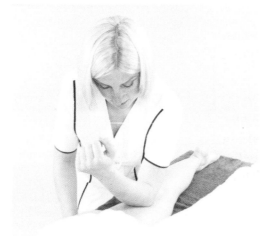

Figure 6.7b NMT

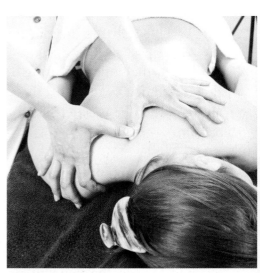

Note

If the pain increases as the trigger point is worked, this may be a sign of inflammation so the pressure should instantly be released.

Figure 6.7c NMT

the sensations of pain felt there. This may cause discomfort for the client, so when applying pressure ask the client to state a number between one and three: one, if the pressure is too little; two, if the pressure if just right; and three, if the pressure is too much. Adjust the pressure accordingly.

The therapist should use massage movements to stretch the affected muscle after treating it and should not give further neuromuscular treatment for 48 hours.

Effects of neuromuscular massage

◆ Relieves pain.

◆ Increases blood circulation therefore aids healing.

◆ Increases output of endorphins, which are the body's own mood-lifting and pain-relieving hormones.

◆ Relieves congestion in nerve pathways.

◆ Improves mobility of joints.

A painful area of the body, such as in a muscle, may sometimes be traced back to one of the main spinal nerves. If the pain is referred, the origin of the pain may be within a spinal nerve and working that specific spinal nerve will help to ease the discomfort. Each spinal nerve divides into branches, forming groups of nerves called plexuses. An example of a plexus is the brachial plexus, which supplies the whole of the shoulders and arms. See Chapter 2.

Another type of neuromuscular technique involves working on specific motor points of muscles, which are deeply massaged with the fingertips. A motor point is where the nerve enters the belly of the muscle. Pressure is applied on a painful or weak muscle but only for about 10 seconds.

Lymphatic drainage massage

Lymphatic drainage massage techniques consist of using gentle and rhythmic hand movements. It is a superficial massage that aids lymphatic drainage. It is thought that applying pressure to superficial lymph vessels will have an effect on the deeper lymph vessels. However, all massage will stimulate the lymphatic flow and so aid drainage. Clients with areas of oedema (fluid retention), commonly seen around the ankles, will benefit from this type of massage as the lymphatic drainage techniques will help to reduce puffiness and remove excess fluid from the affected area.

Lymphatic drainage massage also acts on the body's autonomic nervous system and has a calming effect on the sympathetic nerves. Therefore clients find the treatment very relaxing.

This massage consists of using the tips of fingers or thumbs and applying varying pressures according to the area being treated, although deep pressure is not required. Long, gentle strokes will help gently to push lymph towards the nearest lymph gland. Short, pumping strokes may also be used.

Contra-indications to lymphatic drainage massage

Lymphatic drainage massage should not be used on clients suffering with the following conditions, unless their doctor advises that treatment may go ahead:

- cancer
- lymphoedema
- heart and circulatory problems
- kidney problems
- diabetes.

Also, see contra-indications for body massage in Chapter 3.

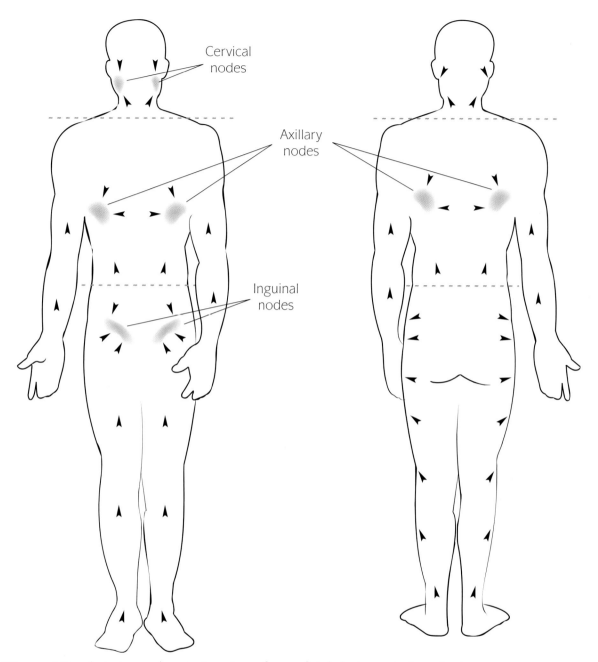

Figure 6.8 *Anterior and posterior view of superficial drainage in lymphatic system*

Cervical nodes

Axillary nodes

Inguinal nodes

Note

To help with fluid retention around the ankles, elevate the legs while the client is lying on the couch to a maximum of 45 degrees.

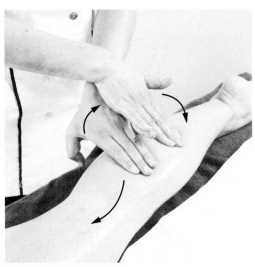

Figure 6.9a *Pumping to lower leg*

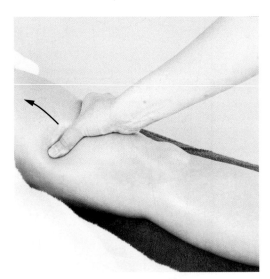

Figure 6.9b *Pumping to thigh*

Effects of lymphatic drainage massage

◆ Increases lymphatic circulation.

◆ Increases blood circulation.

◆ Helps to speed up removal of waste products from muscles.

◆ Reduces build up of excess fluid.

◆ Promotes relaxation.

Some examples of lymphatic drainage techniques follow.

1 Pumping (stride standing)
Using the index, middle and ring fingers of each hand, alternately stroke and push an area with the fingers. Use a gentle pumping action and pressure, working towards a group of lymph nodes.

Alternatively, place the hand on to the area to be treated, keeping fingers together and abduct the thumb. Push, pump and then release pressure and repeat these movements working over the whole area towards the group of lymph nodes.

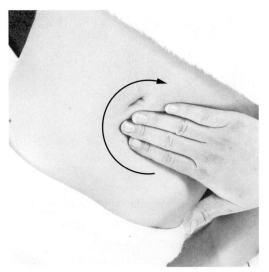

Figure 6.10 *Circles to abdomen*

2 Circles

Place the hand flatly on to the skin, fingers together. Create circles with the fingers ensuring the skin beneath is gently moved. Make sure the fingers are kept straight and work in the direction of lymph nodes. This movement is often used on the lymph node areas. Repeat this movement five times.

3 Side of hands push

With hands flat and fingers together place the little-finger side of the hand on to the skin. Use the whole side of the hands to work towards an area of lymph nodes, as if helping the flow of lymph towards the nodes. The hands can be worked alternately over an area.

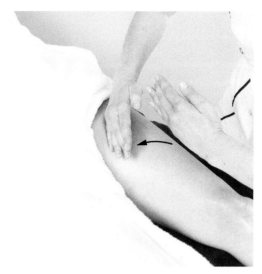

Figure 6.11   *Side of hands push*

Stretching and releasing

Muscle stretching techniques are useful for helping to relax and lengthen tight, contracted muscles. The therapist may apply a stretch to a muscle or the client may be asked to stretch a muscle and the therapist can apply pressure to gain a further stretch. Movements are carried out so that a muscle is taken slowly to the end of its range. The position is held so that the muscle adapts to the stretch and so can then be stretched further. This causes the muscle to relax so the muscle length is increased.

Muscle stretching techniques are beneficial for the following reasons:

- helps to promote relaxation within contracted muscle

- increases elasticity and length of muscles

- improves posture

- increases pressure on a tendon, therefore causes relaxation of the muscle

- improves the circulation so brings nutrients to the area and rids the area of waste products

- stimulates flaccid muscles to help increase their muscle tone

- if performed after exercise, it reduces muscle soreness.

Effleurage or warm up exercises can be used to warm the muscles beforehand and the therapist then gently stretches the tight muscle until there is a mild stretch. There may be a feeling of mild discomfort, however, there should be no pain. The stretch should be held for 10 seconds and then released for 2 seconds to relax fully, and slowly and steadily stretched further in this position and held comfortably for

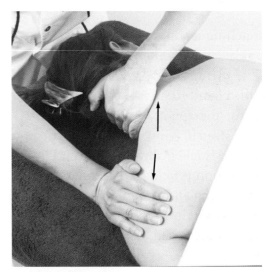

Figure 6.12 *Stretch and release to neck*

These movements are carried out as the client exhales.

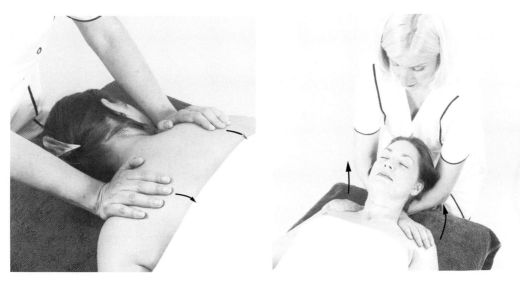

Figure 6.13 *Stretch and release to trapezius muscle*

another 10 seconds. The movements should be smooth and controlled. Over time the stretch can be increased and held for 20–30 seconds.

If there is an imbalance, some muscles may be weak and others strong and tight. To restore balance it is necessary to stretch the tight muscles first and allow the weak muscles to be strengthened.

Shiatsu

Shiatsu originates from Japan and means 'finger pressure'. It involves using pressures

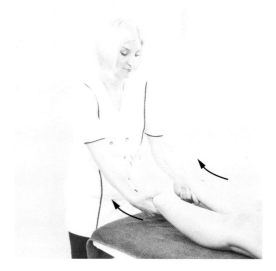

Figure 6.14 *Stretch and release to hamstrings*

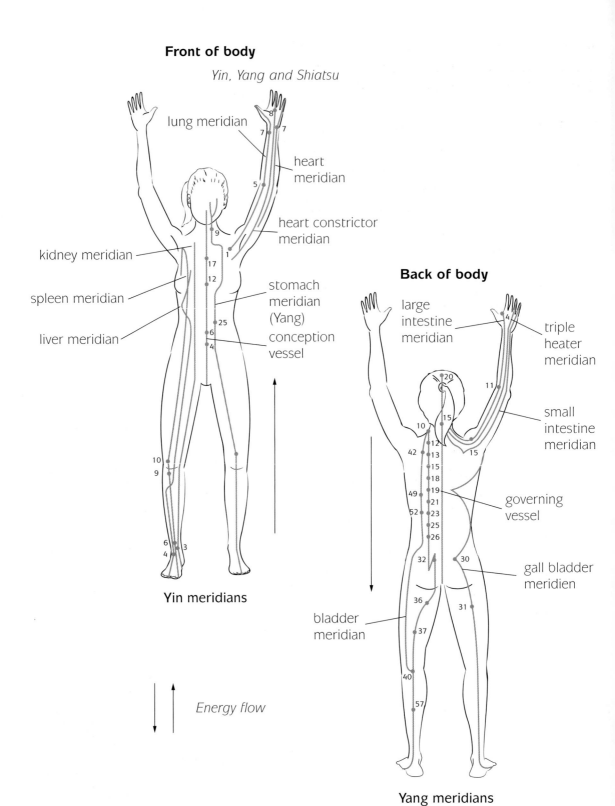

Figure 6.15 *Meridians of the body*

on certain points of the body (the same as used in acupuncture). It can be carried out through clothing with the client lying on the floor.

The fingers, thumbs, palms, elbows and knees can all be used when giving shiatsu treatment and help to aid the smooth flow of energy through the body, known as ki. Ki is vital as it supports, nourishes and protects emotional and physical well-being. Ki is said to pass through 12 main channels or meridians in the body. When in good health energy flows smoothly through the meridians. If ki becomes blocked, for example by negative thoughts, it may cause stress and ill health. Holding and applying pressure to points

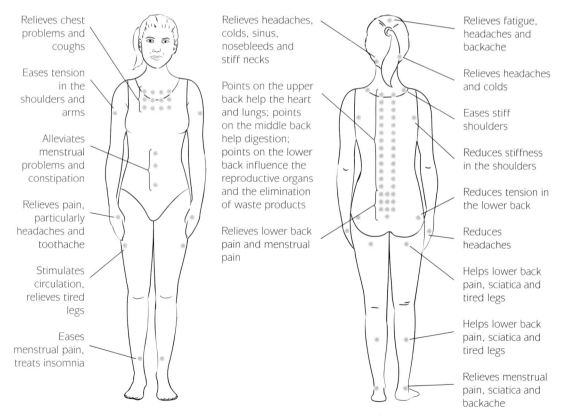

Relieves chest problems and coughs

Eases tension in the shoulders and arms

Alleviates menstrual problems and constipation

Relieves pain, particularly headaches and toothache

Stimulates circulation, relieves tired legs

Eases menstrual pain, treats insomnia

Relieves headaches, colds, sinus, nosebleeds and stiff necks

Points on the upper back help the heart and lungs; points on the middle back help digestion; points on the lower back influence the reproductive organs and the elimination of waste products

Relieves lower back pain and menstrual pain

Relieves fatigue, headaches and backache

Relieves headaches and colds

Eases stiff shoulders

Reduces stiffness in the shoulders

Reduces tension in the lower back

Reduces headaches

Helps lower back pain, sciatica and tired legs

Helps lower back pain, sciatica and tired legs

Relieves menstrual pain, sciatica and backache

Figure 6.16 *Acupressure points of the body*

(known as tsubos) on the meridians can stimulate the ki energy, and help to relieve pain and encourage the body to heal itself.

Acupressure

Shiatsu is a form of acupressure. Acupressure is an ancient Chinese healing method and is helpful to relieve pain and promote good health. It involves applying pressures with

Task 6.3

Use the information on other forms of massage treatment given above to complete Table 6.3.

Table 6.3 Types of massage treatment

Type of massage treatment	Brief description
Deep tissue massage	
Neuromuscular techniques	
Manual lymphatic drainage	
Stretching and releasing	
Shiatsu	
Acupressure	

fingers or thumbs to certain points of the body to help aid the flow of energy, known as chi in China.

By stimulating specific points located along the meridians, acupressure can help restore balance by releasing blocked energy, relieve muscular tensions and also aid the circulation of the blood. These pressure points are the places where the channels come near to the body's surface; therefore it is possible to influence the chi. Acupressure can help many conditions, including headaches, insomnia, depression, colds and digestive disorders. Each acupressure point can be pressed for between one and three minutes. The pressure is applied gradually.

MECHANICAL MASSAGE

Machines can be used to carry out mechanical massage and can either be incorporated in a normal body massage routine or used as a treatment alone. Using this type of equipment will help to prevent overuse of hands and joints, which can result in conditions developing such as repetitive strain injury. Mechanical massage may be carried out using gyratory vibrators, percussion vibrators or audiosonic vibrators.

Gyratory vibrators

There are two main types of gyratory vibrator, the hand-held vibrator and a larger vibrator, often called the G5. There are a variety of heads and attachments that can be used and all have different effects on the body. They are designed to imitate the movements of manual massage. The round and curved sponge heads are similar to effleurage movements, 'the egg box', 'pronged' and 'football' rubber applicators are similar to

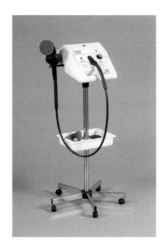

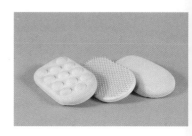

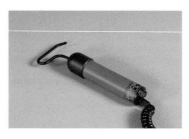

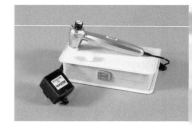

Figure 6.17 *A selection of mechanical massage equipment*

petrissage movements and the heads that are spiky are similar to tapotement movements.

Contra-indications to mechanical massage

- Skin diseases and disorders.
- Thin, elderly, bony clients.
- Recent operations.
- Bruising.
- Varicose veins.
- Over abdomen during menstruation and pregnancy.
- Thrombosis and phlebitis.
- Excessively hairy areas.
- Headaches and migraines if treating the head or face.

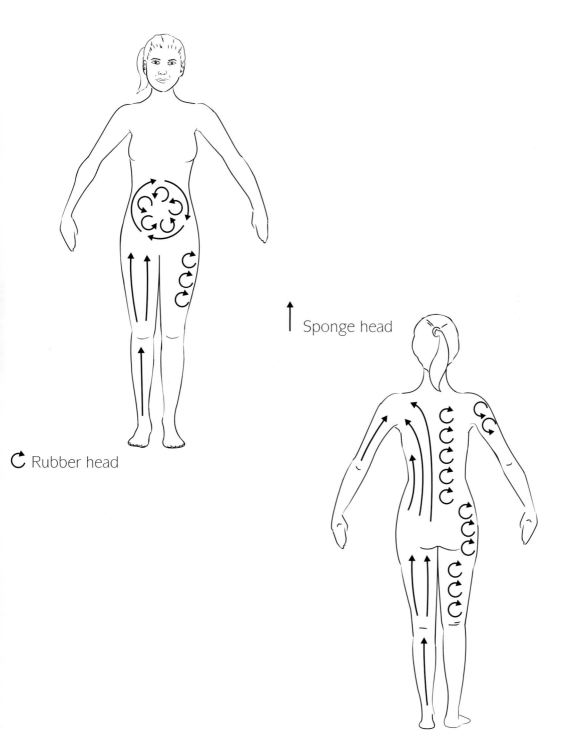

↑ Sponge head

Ↄ Rubber head

Figure 6.18 *Application of strokes when using gyratory vibrator*

Application of strokes when using gyratory vibrators

The order of treatment can be the same as when giving a body massage. When using a gyratory vibrator the strokes can be applied in certain directions over the body. Figure 6.18 shows the direction of strokes that should be used for maximum benefit.

Effects of using gyratory vibrators

- Stimulates blood and lymphatic circulation.
- Helps to relieve pain and tension in muscles.
- Helps to ease areas of contraction in muscle.
- The increased blood circulation and desquamating effect may improve the condition of the skin.
- May cause reddening of the skin.

Percussion vibrator

This is a small piece of machinery that can be easily held in the hand. Its effects are similar to that of tapotement movements. The head quickly moves up and down on the skin and can be fitted with a variety of attachments such as sponge or spike applicators. They are used mainly on the shoulder, neck and face areas, although bony areas should be avoided.

Audiosonic vibrator

This hand-held piece of equipment is ideal to use on small areas. It produces a humming sound and causes sound waves to pass deep into the tissues. It has little effect on the surface of the skin so can be used on sensitive areas. It is helpful for treating tension nodules (knots) in muscles and to treat ligaments around joints.

Effects of using audiosonic vibrators

- Increases blood and lymphatic circulation.
- Relieves pain.
- Relaxes tension nodules.
- Aids desquamation so improves the condition of the skin.

1 State **five** reasons why a massage may need to be modified in some way.

....

....

....

....

....

2 Why are mobility exercises helpful for stiff joints?

....

....

....

3 What is the purpose of deep tissue massage?

....

....

....

4 What is the function of lymphatic massage drainage techniques?

....

....

....

5 When would stretching and releasing techniques be used?

....

....

....

6 What is the purpose of neuromuscular massage?

. . . .

. . . .

. . . .

7 What is the purpose of shiatsu and acupressure?

. . . .

. . . .

. . . .

8 Name **3** machines that are used to carry out mechanical massage.

. . . .

. . . .

. . . .

Legislation, Good Practice and Setting Up a Business

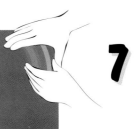

7

It is important to understand the health, safety and hygiene regulations relating to massage treatment. Massage therapists need to be aware of the following legislation and guidelines.

HEALTH AND SAFETY AT WORK ACT 1974

This Act ensures that employers and employees maintain high standards of health and safety in the workplace.

Employers are responsible for the health and safety of anyone who enters their premises. If an employer has more than five employees, the workplace must have a health and safety policy, of which all staff must be aware.

Employers and employees have responsibilities under this Act. Employers must ensure the following:

- The workplace does not pose a risk to the health and safety of employees and clients.

- Protective equipment is provided.

- All equipment must be safe and have regular checks.

- There must be a safe system of cash handling, such as when taking money to the bank.

- Staff should be aware of safety procedures in the workplace, and have the necessary information, instruction and training.

Employees' responsibilities include:

◆ To follow the health and safety policy.

◆ Read the hazards warning labels on containers and follow the advice.

◆ Report any potential hazard such as glass breakage or spillage of chemicals to the relevant person in the workplace.

Task 7.1

When you spot a hazard or error in Figure 7.1 opposite, draw a circle around it.

HEALTH AND SAFETY (FIRST AID) REGULATIONS 1981

A place of work must have a first aid box containing the following: plasters, bandages, wound dressings, safety pins, eyepads and cleaning wipes.

First aid should be carried out by someone who is qualified (ensure you know who is qualified in your place of work). Information such as the patient's name, date, place, time, events, any injury and treatment/advice given must be recorded.

Note

It is recommended that you undertake first aid training for emergency first aid.

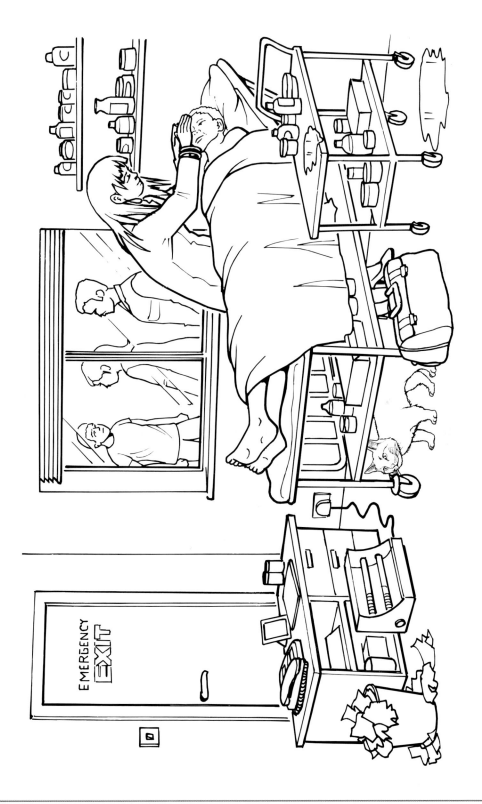

Figure 7.1 *Spot the hazards*

Table 7.1 Basic first aid in the workplace

Problem	First aid procedure
Allergies	If the skin is red, itchy and inflamed after using oil or cream the client may have an allergy. First, remove the product using water. If possible, apply a cold compress or cold pack to reduce any swelling.
Burns	The affected area should be held under a cold, running tap for a while. If the burn is serious, medical attention should be sought, however it can be loosely covered with a sterile dressing in the meantime.
Cuts	Rinse the cut under a running tap. If there is bleeding a sterile gauze or a pad of cotton wool can be placed over the wound. Keep the affected part lifted if possible and apply pressure for a few minutes. Seek medical attention if the bleeding does not stop. Remember to put on disposable gloves as soon as possible before touching the wound.
Dizziness	Persons should be positioned with their head down between their knees. This will help blood to flow to the head.
Electric shock	Person must not be touched until disconnected from the electricity supply. A qualified person can give artificial respiration. Call for an ambulance.
Epilepsy	If a person is having an epileptic fit, remove any items around him or her that could cause injury. Check airway is clear.
Fainting	Lie the person flat, bend the knees and place pillows under the lower legs. This will increase the flow of blood to the head.
Fall	Do not move the person if he or she complains of back or neck pain. Cover him or her with a blanket and call an ambulance.
Nosebleeds	Sit persons in the chair with their head bent forward. Ask them to firmly pinch the soft part of the nose until bleeding stops.
Objects in the eye	Twist a dampened piece of cotton wool or tissue and try to move the object to the inside corner of the eye. Otherwise

FIRE PRECAUTIONS ACT 1971

This Act states that all staff must be trained in fire and emergency evacuation procedure and the premises must have fire escapes.

- There must be adequate fire-fighting equipment in good working order.
- Clearly marked fire exit doors should remain unlocked and must not be obstructed.
- Smoke alarms must be used and regularly checked.
- All staff must be trained in fire drill procedures and this information should be displayed at the workplace.

Fire extinguishers

Fire extinguishers are colour coded for different types of fire. Table 7.2 states the colour, contents and for what type of fire the extinguishers are used.

Table 7.2 Types of fire extinguishers

Colour of label	Contents of fire extinguisher	Type of fire it is used for
Red	Water	Wood, paper, clothing and plastics.
Blue	Dry powder	Electrical fires, oils, alcohols, solvents, paint. Flammable liquids and gases. (Not on chip or fat pan fires.)
Cream	Foam	Flammable liquids. Do not use for electrical fires.
Black	Carbon dioxide (CO_2)	For use on electrical fires but switch off electrical supply first. Grease, fats, oils, paint, flammable liquids. (Not on chip or fat pan fires.)
Green	Vapourising liquids	Electrical fires, flammable liquids.

Fire blankets are used to put out fires such as chip pan fires. The blanket covers the fire and helps prevent oxygen from fuelling the flames and so the fire is put out.

CONTROL OF SUBSTANCES HAZARDOUS TO HEALTH (COSHH) 1994

COSHH covers substances used in practice which can cause ill health. Hazardous substances such as oils must be used and stored away safely. All containers that contain potentially harmful chemicals must be clearly labelled. Manufacturers often give safety information regarding their products.

Corrosive

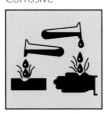

Oxidising

Toxic

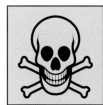

Harmful irritant

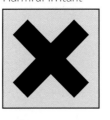

Highly flammable

Explosive

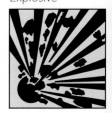

Figure 7.2 *Hazard symbols*

ELECTRICITY AT WORK ACT 1989

This Act is concerned with safety while using electricity. Any electrical equipment must be checked regularly to ensure it is safe. All checks should be listed in a record book and would be important evidence in case of any legal action.

REPORTING OF INJURIES, DISEASES AND DANGEROUS OCCURRENCES REGULATIONS (RIDDOR) 1995

Minor accidents should be entered into a record book, stating what occurred and what action was taken. Ideally all concerned should sign. If as a result of an accident at work anyone is off work for more than three days, or someone is seriously injured, has a type of occupational disease certified by the doctor, or even dies, then the employer should send a report to the local authority environmental health department as soon as possible.

MANUAL HANDLING OPERATIONS REGULATIONS 1992

Incorrect lifting and carrying of goods can result in injuries such as back injury. Employers must assess the risks to their employees and make sure they provide training if necessary.

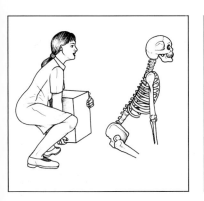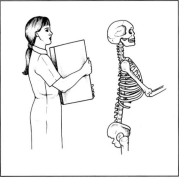

Figure 7.3 *When lifting, keep your knees bent and your back straight at all time to avoid injury*

LOCAL GOVERNMENT ACT 1982

By-laws are laws made by your local council and are primarily concerned with hygiene practice. Different councils around the UK will have different by-laws. You will probably find there is not a by-law relating to massage treatment in your area. However, advice can be sought by contacting your local environmental health officer.

LOCAL GOVERNMENT (MISCELLANEOUS PROVISIONS) ACT 1982

A therapist must apply for a licence from the local environmental health and trading standards department if needles are used for any treatments such as acupuncture or ear piercing.

PERFORMING RIGHTS

Some therapists like to play relaxing music while giving a massage treatment. Any music played in waiting or treatment rooms is termed a public performance. If you play music you may need to purchase a licence from Phonographic Performance Ltd (PPL) or from the Performing Rights Society (PRS). These organisations collect the licence fees and give money to the performer and record companies. If you do not buy a licence legal action may be taken against you.

However, many composers of music are not members of the PPL or PRS so no fee will need to be paid. To find out if you will need a licence contact the supplier of the music.

DATA PROTECTION ACT 1998

Any information about an individual such as a client that is stored on to a computer must be registered with the Data Protection Register. This Act ensures that information is used by the therapist only and not given to anyone else without the client's permission. This Act does not apply to records stored manually, such as record cards stored in boxes.

CONSUMER PROTECTION ACT 1987

This Act provides the customer with protection when purchasing goods or services to ensure that products are safe for use on the client during the treatment, or are safe to be sold as a retail product.

In the past if a person was injured they had to prove that the manufacturer was negligent before they could sue for damages. This Act removed the need to prove negligence. A customer can sue a supplier without having to prove they were negligent.

COSMETIC PRODUCTS (SAFETY) REGULATIONS 1996

These relate to the Consumer Protection Act 1987 and require that cosmetics and toiletries are tested and safe for use.

TRADE DESCRIPTIONS ACTS 1968 AND 1972

A description of a product or service, either spoken or written, must be accurate. It is illegal to use false or misleading descriptions to sell, e.g. state a product can cure a skin disorder, if this information is inaccurate.

Note

A product should be sold at its full price for at least 28 days before a reduced price can be offered.

SALE AND SUPPLY OF GOODS ACT 1994 (REPLACED THE SALES OF GOODS AND SERVICES ACT 1982)

This Act identifies the contract, which takes place between the seller (therapist) and the customer (client) when a product is purchased. This Act makes the seller responsible for ensuring that the goods are of good merchantable quality. It covers all goods, even those used as part of the treatment. It requires that the person giving the service must do so with reasonable care and skill, within a reasonable time and for a reasonable charge.

Sex Discrimination Acts 1975, 1986 and the Race Relations Act 1976

The Equal Opportunities Commission investigates complaints alleging discrimination against job applicants because of their sex, race or marital status.

Protection of Children Act 1999

Employers involved in the care of children (anyone under 18 years old) should check the names of people they intend to employ to ensure they are not included in a list called the Consultancy Index List. This list contains names of individuals considered unsuitable to work with children.

Codes of Practice and Codes of Ethics

Industry Codes of Practice for Hygiene in Salons and Clinics

The Vocational Training Charitable Trust in association with the Federation of Holistic Therapists publishes the code of practice. The code of practice is concerned with hygiene in the salon and gives guidelines for the therapist. Local by-laws also contain these guidelines to ensure good hygienic practice and avoid cross-infection.

Industry Code of Ethics

A code of ethics is a set of guidelines, which a professional massage therapist must ensure that they follow.

- All health, safety and hygiene legislation must be adhered to and the therapist should be adequately insured.
- The best possible treatment is given to the client.
- The client is respected and dignity is maintained at all times.
- Never claim to cure a condition.

- Do not treat a client who is contra-indicated to treatment.

- All clients are treated in a professional manner regardless of their colour, sex or religion.

- All information given, written or verbal, is confidential and should not be disclosed to anyone without written permission, except when required to do so by law.

- Records of treatments carried out are up to date and complete.

- Further training is undertaken to enhance skills.

- Become a member of a professional massage association.

INSURANCE

Employers Liability (Compulsory Insurance) Act 1969

Employers must take out insurance policies in case of claims by employees for injury, disease or illness related to the workplace. It protects an employer against any claims made by an employee.

A certificate must be displayed at work to show that the employer has this insurance.

- **Public liability insurance**: this insurance protects you if a client or member of the public becomes injured on your premises, for example if they fall off the couch.

- **Product liability insurance**: this type of insurance protects you against claims arising from products used by clients.

- **Treatment liability insurance**: this insurance protects you in the event of a claim arising from malpractice. It covers the practitioner for damage to clients caused by the treatment itself.

In Table 7.3 below, write a brief description of each piece of legislation and type of insurance.

Table 7.3 Legislation and guidelines

Legislation/guidelines	Brief description
Health and Safety at Work Act 1974	
Health and Safety (First Aid) Regulations 1981	
Fire Precautions Act 1971	
COSHH 1994	
Electricity at Work Act 1989	
RIDDOR 1995	

Table 7.3 Continued

Legislation/guidelines	Brief description
Manual Handling Operations Regulations 1992	
Local Government Act 1982	
Local Government (Miscellaneous Provisions) Act 1982	
Performing Rights	
Data Protection Act 1998	
Consumer Protection Act 1987	
Cosmetic Products (Safety) Regulations 1996	

Table 7.3 Continued

Legislation/guidelines	Brief description
Trade Descriptions Acts 1968 and 1972	
Sale and Supply of Goods Act 1994	
Sex Discrimination Acts 1975, 1986 and Race Relations Act 1976	
Protection of Children Act 1999	
Employers Liability (Compulsory Insurance) Act 1969	
Public liability insurance	

Table 7.3 Continued

Legislation/guidelines	Brief description
Product liability insurance	
Treatment liability insurance	

BUSINESS PLAN

If you intend to set up a business the following information will help you to prepare a business plan.

Research

- ◆ Research local competition. How much do they charge for treatments? What are their hours of business?

- ◆ Research the prices of products and equipment that you will need to start your business.

- ◆ How will you advertise and maintain public relations? How much will advertising your business cost?

- ◆ Carry out market research in the area in which you propose to run your business. Are people interested in the services you have to offer?

- ◆ Will you be self-financed or will you require external finance, such as taking out a loan? Maybe seek the professional advice of an accountant.

Note

Banks will give you professional advice regarding setting up a business.

- What insurance policies will you need to take out, and how much will such policies cost?

- Research what is meant by the terms 'freehold' and 'leasehold'.

- Will you rent a room; how much will you pay?

- Will you run a mobile business? What costs are involved?

- Research all health, safety and hygiene issues and cost these in also if necessary.

- Consider the catchment area; who are you trying to attract and from where?

- If you take over an existing business, what improvement could you make?

Treatment room

- What are the considerations when choosing a treatment room? For example, is there room for clients to park or will there be passing trade?

- Draw a plan of your treatment room; what colour scheme will you choose and what equipment and resources will you need?

Clients and services

- How will you ensure client satisfaction so that the client returns for future treatments?

- How much will you charge clients for each treatment? How long will each treatment take? You will need to ensure the treatments are cost effective.

- How will you ensure you maximise profitability, e.g. timekeeping, minimise wastage, etc?

- Will you require staff?

Note

It is a good idea to design a price list, and any other leaflet, which gives a brief outline of the services you will provide.

1 Which Act ensures that employers and employees maintain high standards of health and safety in the workplace?

   ....

2 Which Act states that smoke alarms must be used and fire exit doors should remain unlocked and unobstructed?

   ....

3 Which fire extinguisher would you use if there was a fire caused by paper or clothing?

   ....

4 Which legislation states that hazardous substances such as oils must be stored safely?

   ....

5 Which Act ensures that client information stored on computer must be registered with the Data Protection Register?

   ....

6 What is the purpose of the Code of Ethics?

   ....

7 Why is it important to take out insurance if you are working as a massage therapist?

   ....

8
Examination Preparation

MULTIPLE CHOICE QUESTIONS

These multiple choice questions will help you to prepare for body massage examinations. Decide which is the correct answer and put a circle around either (a), (b), (c) or (d).

1   Massage has been recorded in China as early as:

(a)   8000 BC

(b)   3000 BC

(c)   AD 120

(d)   AD 500

2   In the 16th century Ambroise Pare (1517–90) graded massage into the following types:

(a)   soft, average and hard

(b)   soft, medium and rapid

(c)   gentle, average and quick

(d)   gentle, medium and vigorous

3   Which Swedish physiologist developed 'Swedish massage'?

(a)   Po Henrick Lang

(b)   Pa Henrick Leng

(c)   Per Henrick Ling

(d)   Pu Henrick Lang

4   The word 'massage' is thought to have derived from which Arabic word meaning to 'press softly'?

(a)   *mass'h*

(b)   *mesh'h*

(c)   *mush'h*

(d)   *mish'h*

5   Which of the following is *not* a benefit of massage treatment?

(a)   improves digestion

(b)   relieves stiffness in joints

(c)   will mend a fractured bone

(d)   relaxes the mind and body

6   Which of the following conditions is *not* a stress related problem?

(a)   eczema

(b)   headaches

(c)   indigestion

(d)   scabies

7   Slow, deep and rhythmic breathing triggers responses in the body including which of the following?

(a)   increased heart rate

(b) slower heart rate

(c) causes increased amounts of adrenalin to be released

(d) decreases the amount of oxygen delivered to cells

8   Meditation can help trigger responses in the body. Which of the following is *not* a response caused by meditating?

(a) relaxation of tense muscles

(b) regulation of breathing rate

(c) lower blood pressure

(d) increased anxiety levels

9   Which of the following is *not* an effect that massage has on the skin?

(a) stimulation of sebaceous glands

(b) desquamation of the skin

(c) sweat glands become less active

(d) increased blood circulation

10   Which of the following is an effect that massage has on the skeletal system?

(a) stimulates blood flow to the periosteum, increasing the supply of nutrients

(b) causes the bones to become more rigid

(c) decreases the amount of calcium stored within bones

(d) causes the bones to enlarge

11   Which of the following is *not* an effect that massage has on the muscular system?

(a) increases blood supply, bringing oxygen and nutrients

(b) helps to make muscles bulkier and larger

(c) helps to break down nodules

(d) helps to relax muscles that are tense

12   Which of the following is *not* an effect that massage has on the cardiovascular system?

(a) causes reduction in red blood cell production

(b) produces erythema

(c) stimulates blood flow

(d) aids venous return

13   Which of the following is an effect that massage has on the lymphatic system?

(a) decreases the amount of fat transported

(b) lowers resistance to infection

(c) causes an increase in the amount of lymph nodes

(d) helps with fluid retention

14   Which of the following is *not* a contra-indication to massage?

(a) chloasma

(b) high blood pressure

(c) bone fracture

(d) thrombosis

15   Which of the following is a postural fault?

(a) psychosis

(b) poliosis

(c) lordosis

(d) psoriasis

16 Which of the following is *not* a use of effleurage?

(a) to warm the skin, prior to deeper massage

(b) to interlink massage movements

(c) to break down fatty tissue

(d) to help spread the massage medium

17 Which of the following massage movements is a type of petrissage?

(a) kneading

(b) hacking

(c) stroking

(d) shaking

18 Which of the following is *not* a use of petrissage?

(a) helps to relieve stiffness and pain in muscles

(b) helps to relieve constipation

(c) stimulates poor blood circulation

(d) helps to promote oedema

19 Which of the following massage movements is a type of tapotement?

(a) vibrations

(b) beating

(c) effleurage

(d) knuckling

20 Which of the following is *not* a use of tapotement?

(a) to improve the blood circulation

(b) to improve the lymphatic circulation

(c) to promote relaxation

(d) to improve muscular tone

21 Tapotement massage movements should *not* be used on?

(a) bony areas

(b) fleshy areas

(c) clients wanting a stimulating massage

(d) people with poor muscle tone

22 Friction comes from the Latin word *fricare*, meaning to?

(a) rub

(b) pinch

(c) stroke

(d) pick up

23 If a client has come for a relaxing massage, which of the following massage movements would be omitted?

(a) effleurage

(b) tapotement

(c) petrissage

(d) stroking

24 What is erythema?

(a) a type of massage movement

(b) tension within muscle

(c) a type of blood cell

(d) redness of the skin

25 What is cellulite?

(a) subcutaneous fat causing dimpling of the skin

(b) an allergic reaction

(c) a substance that damages tissues

(d) a layer of the skin

26 Which of the following is *not* a type of medium commonly used in massage?

(a) vegetable oil

(b) talc

(c) mineral oil

(d) cream

27 Which of the following pre-heat treatments involves the use of a lamp?

(a) sauna

(b) infra-red

(c) steam bath

(d) paraffin wax

28 Palpation involves which of the following?

(a) feeling or sensing the changes in tissues

(b) blending the oils

(c) manipulating the muscle tissue

(d) using machines to carry out massage

29 Excluding a consultation, a back massage will usually take what length of time?

(a) 30 minutes

(b) 20 minutes

(c) 10 minutes

(d) 40 minutes

30 A contra-action is also known as a?

(a) contra-indication

(b) mobility exercise

(c) postural exercise

(d) healing crisis

31 Which of the following is *not* a contra-action to massage treatment?

(a) tiredness

(b) erythema

(c) minor bleeding

(d) aching/soreness in muscles

32 Which of the following aftercare advice would be given to clients?

(a) smoke lots of cigarettes

(b) drink lots of water

(c) do some vigorous exercise

(d) eat large meals

33 What is oedema?

(a) excess fat

(b) a bone disease

(c) an infectious skin disorder

(d) fluid retention

34 Mobility exercises are carried out to help what?

(a) break down fat

(b) disperse knots

(c) lose weight

(d) loosen stiff joints

35 Which of the following is *not* a machine used to carry out mechanical massage?

(a) gyratory vibrator

(b) percussion vibrator

(c) audiosonic vibrator

(d) ultrasound vibrator

36 If your client had an allergy to an oil what action would you take?

(a) continue to massage

(b) remove the product using water

(c) add more oil to the skin

(d) bandage the area and apply a hot compress

37 If a client fainted, what immediate action would you take?

(a) give them a glass of water

(b) try to stand them up

(c) lie them flat and place a pillow under the lower legs

(d) sit them in a chair

38 For what do the initials COSHH stand?

(a) control of substances hurtful to health

(b) control of substances helpful to health

(c) control of situations hazardous to health

(d) control of substances hazardous to health

39 Which of the following would you *not* find contained within a fire extinguisher?

(a) water

(b) petrol

(c) carbon dioxide

(d) foam

40 Health and safety relating directly to employers and employees is the subject of which Act of Parliament?

(a) Health and Safety at Work Act 1974

(b) Consumer Protection Act 1987

(c) RIDDOR

(d) Data Protection Act 1998

Index

Note: Entries in *italics* denote figures
Entries in **bold** denote tables